A-B-C-D-Ease of Healthy Eating For Life…Lose Weight Too

By John Mayes

FIRST EDITION - FIRST PRINTING

Library of Congress Control Number: 2003113419
ISBN#: 1-56411-276-4
YBBG#: 0297

Cover photo by: Ron Contarsy

Published in the U. S. A.
By
CONQUERING BOOKS, L.L.C.
210 East Arrowhead Drive #1
Charlotte, N. C. 28213
(704) 509-2226
www.conqueringbooks.com

ACKNOWLEDGEMENT

My thanks to my family who provided me with support with the writing of this book. It was a dream come true which started with my wife, Veronica, in our young tender years. She helped me select the career in Nutrition and Health Care Administration. Thank you so much for your support. Tyron, my son, thanks for the beautiful photography work and creativity. My son, Todd, shared my hopes and dreams and his support was invaluable. My special thanks to Anthony Recanitini, who attended the school of visual arts, for providing most of the beautiful art work for the book. I look forward to working with him again. My deep appreciation to the models in the book, Diann Sprosty, Jo-Ann Vasta and Brian Brown. Special thanks to Eduicael Dator and Judy Birmingham for their expertise in helping to put the book together. To all my friends, thanks so much for your ongoing encouragement for me to complete the book. I am extremely grateful to all my family and friends for their excitement, ongoing support, and to all my deepest love and appreciation.

CONTENTS

	Page
Introduction	1

Section A   18
This is the beginning, the starting point to help you jump start
an easy, healthy eating regimen for life and lose weight too.
Dieting does not work.

Section B   80
This section supports what you have learned and what you
have put into motion.

Section C   110
This section plays a primary role in showing you how to get
rid of some of the old and opening the doors for some of the new.

Section D   141
You cannot get too much of good, healthy information, more is
better. Enjoy eating healthier without giving up taste.

Section E – PART I   194
A light exercise program is a must during weight loss. This will
help you lose weight, burn fat, and tone the body.

Section E – PART II   232
Everything leading to this section is actually showing you how
easy it is to eat healthy and lose weight too. This section will
provide you with additional information that will aid in weight
loss and body toning.

INTRODUCTION

The information in this book that will show you how to eat healthy for life, lose weight, and maintain your weight without dieting. I hope that this book will inspire you to get off the dieting craze and keep yourself healthy primarily through healthier habits.

Almost everyone that has been dieting for long periods of time can control him or herself and create a better and healthier lifestyle. I have mapped out the easiest way for you to take responsibilities for the way you view food. With this knowledge, you will have important information available to make easy daily changes. It is my goal to provide you with the necessary information for you to stay healthier longer and also lose weight and keep it off. You are responsible for your well being, how do you value your life?

A total healthy lifestyle should be as natural as brushing your teeth. Only a very few fraction of percentage of our health and weight problem is attributable to genetic and biochemistry.

For most of us what our problem is for being unhealthy or obese is consequently due to unhealthy lifestyle, lack of exercise, chronic stress, lack of proper sleep, exposure to toxins, poor nutrients intake, and just plain overeating.

You can eat healthier, lose weight and maintain your weight within a healthy range for you without counting calories or fat grams. Stop the dieting syndrome.

YOU DON'T NEED WILLPOWER TO LOSE WEIGHT

It does not take will power to lose weight, you will only be setting yourself for failure. When it comes to food intake and weight loss, the only willpower you need is knowledge. The first step to weight loss is to learn how to eat healthy. I am not too concerned about the amount of food you consume, but the type of food you buy and how you prepare it. Lower-fat cooking and eating is the first key to weight loss. You can eat the same amount of food and still lose weight. This will prevent fat craving and stop hunger caused from very low-fat calorie dieting. In time, you will learn how to cut out additional calories and not get hungry by healthy snacking and with the consumption of ice cold water. Your body has a natural fat burning system that acts like a furnace. You will, at times, be able to eat more and still lose weight. How is this possible? It may take more than seven to eight times as many calories to turn a food that's rich in complex carbohydrates into body fat as it does to turn dietary fat into body fat. The body better recognizes dietary fat and requires less work.

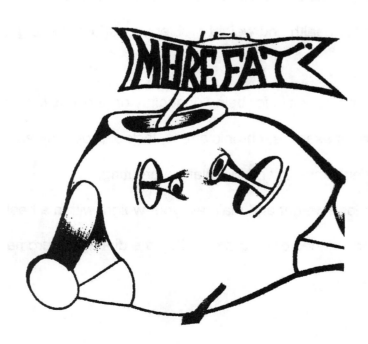

WHAT IF YOUR WEIGHT IS ALWAYS IN THE NORMAL RANGE? WHY EAT LOWER FAT? WHY EXERCISE/OR INCREASE PHYSICAL ACTIVITY?

You should always eat healthy. By eating lower-fat meals more often with the proper balance of physical exercise/activity, you will help yourself maintain your weight as you get older and will help prevent unwanted illness.

The following are some benefits to a healthy lifestyle:

- Feel better

- Look healthier

- Lower blood pressure

- Less depression

- Unclog arteries (lower cholesterol)

- Reduce risk of some types of cancer

- Improve immune system

- More energy

- Help prevent male impotence

- Improve bone fracture in females

YOUR BODY CAN BE A FAT BURNING FURNACE

Our body loves fat. Mother Nature programmed us this way. The body prefers to store fat for fuel. The body stores fat easier and it take longer to burn. It is extremely hard to lose fat because our body craves fat. Our forefathers were able to consume larger amounts of fat and burn it off because of the harder type of work. The extra fat calories were burned off easy. Our ancestors needed the extra fat because they often went days without eating; the excess fat was required to help maintain a more normal weight. With the changing times, the excess fat intake is not needed. We can control our body's natural fat-burning system and use it as a furnace to burn the excess fat that is not needed.

SETPOINT

It is believed that there is a setting inside our body that regulates our weight. This setting is called the "setpoint." The body defends this setting tenaciously. If you persist with a low calorie diet, the body lowers its metabolic rate so that you burn fewer calories. You will stop losing weight unless you change your setpoint. You can begin to start losing weight by changing or resetting your setpoint by exercising. You do not need an enormous amount of exercise. Moderate exercise will burn up calories and speed up the rate at which calories are burned.

- Bicycling
- Walking (brisk)
- Dancing
- Jogging
- Jumping
- Jumping rope
- Swimming

Healthy meal plan, exercise, activity, and behavior modifications are still the mainstay of long-term weight control. Some researchers are studying drugs that appear to burn fat, regardless of what is eaten or how much. These studies are still in their early stages but there are some herbs that help burn off fat and appear to replace it with muscle tissue.

HAZARDS OF OBESITY

Excessive weight is closely associated with cardiovascular disease, problems with the circulatory system, diabetes, renal disease, gallbladder disease, degenerative arthritis, and gout.

- **HEART:** Obese people more often have heart disease. A reduction in weight may be necessary to relieve strain on the heart or to prevent any further damage to the organ, if any occurred. Obesity may cause: a) irregular heartbeat; b) increased resting heart rate; c) enlarged heart; d) elevated blood pressure; e) increased risk of congestive heart failure.

- **CIRCULATORY SYSTEM:** Obesity is linked to problems of the circulatory system. People with cardiovascular disease should maintain their weight within normal range. This will lessen the work of the heart and circulatory system. In obesity: a) in the blood there is an increase in the levels of cholesterol, triglycerides, ketones, insulin, and reduced level of good cholesterol; b) the risk of arteriosclerosis is greater and there may be inflammation of the veins and there is an increase incidence of essential hypertension.

- **DIABETES:** Most adult diabetics are overweight. People that are potential diabetics should maintain weight within normal range to prevent or to delay the development of the disease. Normal or slightly underweight people are less likely to develop diabetes.

- **KIDNEYS:** It is important to maintain weight as normal as possible. With kidney disorder, there is an increased incidence of hypertension.

- **GALLBLADDER:** Many people with gallbladder disease are overweight. In obese people, there is also an increased risk of gallbladder cancer.

- **PANCREAS:** In the obese person, there is increased incidence of carcinoma (cancer). Any serious disturbances which interfere with the production of a sufficient amount of insulin may lead to diabetes.

- **COLON:** There is a higher incidence of colon cancer in the obese individual. Intestinal mobility may also be decreased.

- **STOMACH:** There is also a higher risk of carcinoma.

- **LUNGS:** In the obese person, respiratory problems are increased due to hyperventilation. Pickwickian Syndrome – an inability to exchange gases in the lungs.

- **BRAIN:** In obesity, there is higher incidence of stroke. The risk of cerebral hemorrhage is increased.

- **ARTHRITIS:** Arthritis is a disease of the joints, which is the principle crippler in this country. In obesity, there is increased incidence of osteoarthritis (a degenerative joint disease). Weight loss is necessary to reduce the added stress on the joints.

- **GOUT:** In obesity, there is an increased incidence of gout (acute inflammation of the joints). With gout, there is a sudden pain in the large toe, with the pain moving up the leg. The overweight person should lose weight gradually. Rapid weight loss can hasten the occurrence of an attack of gout. It is not advisable to lose weight during an acute attack of gout.

- **SURGERY:** Obese people face an extra risk if surgery is needed. If possible, weight should be lost before elective surgery.

- **PREGNANCY:** The obese pregnant woman is more likely to have complications than a woman who is not overweight. The hazard of childbirth is increased in the presence of excessive adipose tissue. With the increased risk that obesity has during pregnancy, additional stress during pregnancy must be avoided. After the pregnancy, the excess weight should be lost gradually.

- **SPECIAL PROBLEMS WITH OBESITY IN FEMALES:** Obese females exhibit a higher mortality (postmenopausal) from cancer of the gallbladder, biliary passage, breast, cervix, uterus, ovaries, and endometrium.

- **SPECIAL PROBLEMS WITH OBESITY IN MALES:** The obese male has a higher incidence of heart attacks and angina as compared to the leaner male. The number of heart attacks and angina in the obese male is triple than that seen in females. Obese males have a higher mortality from cancer of the colon, rectum, and prostate.

- **OTHER PROBLEMS OF OBESITY:** Excess weight places unnecessary strain on the body, such as fatigue, foot problems, and backache. There may be difficulty in walking due to back pain and the extra weight on the feet. Embarrassment, being sensitive to ridicule and disfigurement may cause emotional and psychological problems. On the other hand, an emotional problem may sometimes be the cause of obesity.

OBESITY AND DEATH:

Being overweight is directly linked to 5 of the leading causes of death (heart disease, diabetes, stroke, arteriosclerosis, and some forms of cancer).

Overweight is one of the most pervasive health risks affecting Americans today, after smoking, which causes an estimated 500,000 deaths each year. Obesity-related conditions are the second leading cause of death in this country, resulting in about 300,000 lives annually.

```
_____500,000
S
  M
   O
    K                        _____300,000
     I
      N           OBESITY              _____200,000
       G          RELATED        A
                  CONDITIONS       L
                                    C
                                     O
                                      H
                                       O
                                        L  RELATED
```

WEIGHT GAIN AND AGE

As we get older, the amount of muscle in our bodies tends to decrease. The percentage of fat to muscle will increase. Many of us become less active as we get older. Metabolism also slows down with age. The amounts of calories we need are decreased. If we continue eating the same amount of calories after age 35, we can gain an extra pound each year. If we ignore these trends, we can easily end up severely overweight by age 50.

BODY FAT LOCATION

More important than the amount of extra weight a person carries, is where it is located. Fat in the hips and thighs are less health-threatening than abdominal fat.

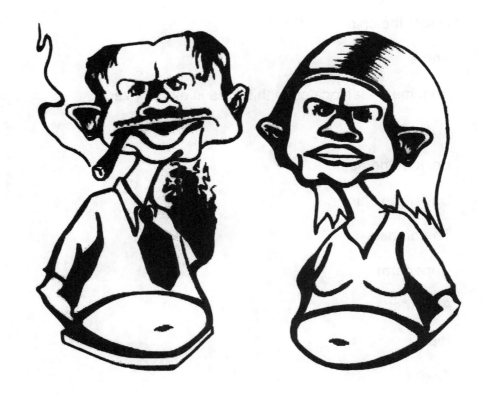

BODY FAT LOCATION

Fat tends to gather in different areas in men and women.

MEN

1. Back of the neck

2. Under the chin

3. Trunk

4. Abdomen – fat located in this area is more hazard

WOMEN

1. Back of the neck

2. Under the chin

3. The breasts

4. Upper arm

5. Abdomen

6. Hips

7. Thighs

8. Buttocks

*Make healthy eating a way of life. The body's basic requirements for calories decrease with age.

DRUGS AND DIET

Buying over the counter drugs or appetite suppressants is not advisable. Some drugs have side effects such as dizziness, nausea, light-headedness, headache, nervousness, weakness, and a false sense of fullness. Due to the false sense of fullness, the patient tends to consume fewer calories, which eventually leads to more serious problems. With prolonged use, it may lead to other problems.

Only a physician should prescribe drug appetite suppressants. He or she will provide regular physicals and blood tests, ensuring that the patient optimum health is maintained. Your nutritionist can work with you to help you plan healthy meals. Dieting does not work.

CRASH DIETS

Crash diets are not recommended unless under the close supervision of a physician or a dietitian. A professional may place a person on a crash diet for a short period of time because the person wants to see quick results. After 7+ days, the person's calories may be increased. Primarily, the person will lose water opposed to fat, while utilizing a crash diet.

For a successful weight loss program, a patient should not lose more than 1 to 2 pounds per week. For example: 2 pounds/week X 52 weeks = 104 pounds per year. Losing weight gradually is safe and more successful than quick weight loss.

The recommended meal plan for weight reduction for women is 1000 to 1200 calories per day. For men, 1500 calories, depending on the activities. Your physician or dietitian must supervise meal plan lower than 1000 calories per day.

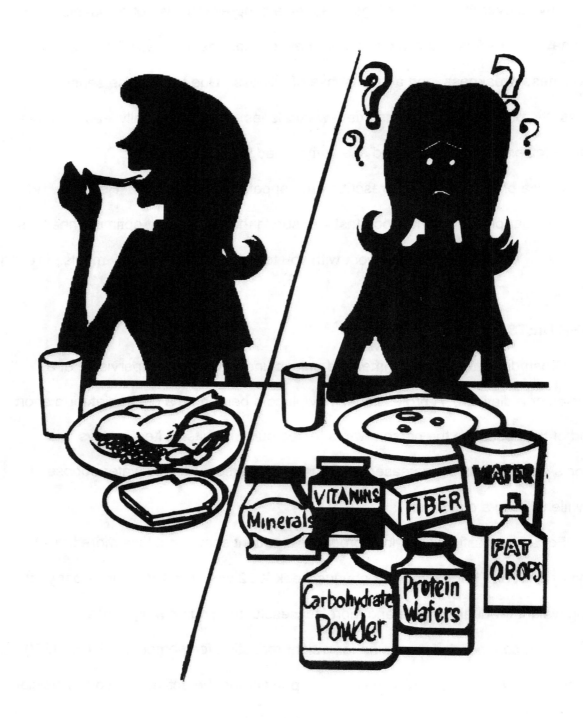

HOW A PERSON GAINS WEIGHT OR BECOMES OVERWEIGHT

- Foods provide heat energy that is measured in units called calories.
  If the amount of energy needed by the body is less than the amount of energy supplied from food, the extra energy will be stored as fat and there will be weight gain.

* The excess fat stored is known as adipose tissue.

TO LOSE WEIGHT

Insufficient energy or calories to meet the needs of the body will cause a decrease in weight. The stored adipose tissue will be used up. You must take in fewer calories and increase your physical activity. Moderate regular exercise along with healthy lower fat meals, keeping variety in mind is the only way.

1. BINGE EATER

You can control your hunger and prevent unhealthy binge eating by eating more often, eat lower fat lower calorie snacks between meals and still lose and maintain weight.

Eating smaller meals throughout the day instead of the regular three meals a day will prevent hunger and will also stabilize the blood sugar level that will cause the body to burn fat more efficiently. So eat more often to prevent over eating at mealtime but choose the right kind of foods that are also high-complex carbohydrate and lower in fat and calories.

2.   THE NIGHT BINGER

They usually start eating heavily at supper and continue to eat throughout the evening and last into the night. They are known as the night refrigerator raiders.

To prevent night bingeing, it is necessary to start eating smaller meals throughout the day with a healthy bedtime snack. The night eater becomes too hungry and when they start eating when they get home at night, the eating is uncontrollable.

After eating supper, have a healthy bedtime snack. This will prevent the nighttime eater from getting too hungry over into the night.

DANGER OF TOO RAPID WEIGHT LOSS

It is not recommended to lose more than 1 to 2 pounds per week. A rapid weight loss should never be attempted without strict medical supervision. Too rapid of a weight loss may result in:

- Dizziness
- Weakness
- Irritability
- Depression
- Problems with the heart
- Problems with other organs
- Skin may wrinkle after a rapid loss of fat
- If the diet is too strict, you are likely to feel uncomfortably hungry.

If you consume 500 calories below your daily energy requirement, you will lose about 1 pound per week or 4 pounds per month. 1000 calories per day below your daily energy requirement, you will lose about 2 pounds per week or 8 pounds per month.

You may not lose exactly at that rate each week, especially for the first week or two. Your water balance, heat loss, metabolism, and your activity influence the amount of weight loss. Your weight loss will average out if you stay on a healthy eating plan. A gradual loss of weight will also give you time to correct your eating habits which will prevent you from regaining the weight you lost.

TEENAGERS AND LOW FAT DIETS

Do not put teenagers on low fat restriction; just let them eat and snack sensibly.

WEIGHING YOURSELF

Weighing yourself is an important part of any weight loss and maintenance program. In a successful weight management regimen, weighing yourself will help you individualize what program is best for you. It will help you plan and meet your weight loss goal. Weighing yourself is important when losing weight accurately. Weighing will help you know if the program is working for you or whether any changes are necessary. I recommend weighing yourself during the weight loss program every 12 to 14 days. During weight maintenance, once a month is enough. During weight maintenance, if your weight goes up more than 5 pounds, review your healthy eating regimen, as needed, and you may also need to increase activity. During weight maintenance, it is not enough to only watch your fat intake. You must also stay active. If you are not active, it will be difficult to maintain your new healthy weight.

YOUR MEASUREMENT AND WEIGHT LOSS

If you find yourself not losing weight at any point in the time during your weight loss program, please do not worry. You are most likely replacing fat tissue with muscle and muscle weighs more than that of fat. You should check your measurements with a tape measure before you start your weight loss program. You will see that you are likely losing inches and becoming leaner.

EMOTIONAL PROBLEMS AND WEIGHT LOSS PROBLEMS

Getting the right kind of professional help is extremely important. Sometimes obesity is linked to emotional problems and makes it a difficult task to lose weight. If this is so, do not be afraid to seek outside help. There are many sources that may help you overcome your obstacles.

The following is a list of professional sources:

1. **Your physician:** Will determine whether there is a physical or mental problem that is causing obesity.

- Check for any serious medical ailments by examination

- Provide personal support

- Refer you to the proper specialist

- Administer medicine, if needed

2. **Psychiatrist or Psychologist:** He or she will determine whether or not there is an emotional problem.

- Provide emotional support

- Refer you to state and local mental health associations, if necessary

- Administer medicine, if needed

3. **Dietitian or Nutritionist:** He or she will create a well-balanced meal plan and exercise plan in which you will lose weight safely.

- They will help you determine your ideal body weight.

- Determine your maintenance caloric level

- Council you on changing your improper eating habits

4. **Nutrition Counselor:** Person trained to lend emotional support while losing weight by helping you to realize what is the root of the problem and by helping you express and come to terms with your problems.

5. **Weight Support Groups:** These individuals or associations should be registered or certified. They provide emotional support by associating with each other during the weight loss and maintenance process.

NOTE: If you do not have a personal physician, call your local hospital for referrals.

SECTION – A

This section is the beginning, the starting point and it will help you to jump start an easy, healthy eating regimen for life. You are provided up front with some powerful information that will aid in improving your total health immediately.

I like to think of Section-A as the beginning of the end. The starting point of eating healthier most of the time and the ending of unnecessary and unhealthy dieting forever.

ARE YOU READY TO START EATING HEALTHY AND LOSE WEIGHT?

Read this section first and you would be able to start eating healthier immediately and this would also help you jumpstart your weight loss. Section A would give you enough information to start eating healthy for life.

The following Sections B, C, D, Ease will support Section A by providing you with a lot of necessary information that will make eating for life easy and fun.

The Ease of eating healthy for life program is not a diet simply because dieting does not work.

You will learn how to burn fat by speeding up your metabolism. You would also find out that you do not need will power to lose weight but what you do need is a little knowledge, okay a little will power will also help.

Although this is not a diet, some people feel that they need to follow a meal plan to lose weight. You have been provided with a variety of meal selections for breakfast, lunch, and dinner. Follow these selections until you feel that you are able to select your own healthy foods, or you can just keep using this guide along with adding your own variety of food to the list. You must add snacks between meals. The calories may be low for your body and if the calories are too low, you will stop losing weight. You must eat enough to keep your metabolic rate up. If you continue dieting, or starving yourself, your metabolism will slow down so much that small portions of food can make you gain weight. You need to eat more often, 5 to 6 smaller meals a day. Your in-between meals (snacks) should be just enough to get you by until your next meal. Switching from one or two large meals per day to five or six smaller meals will help prevent hunger and will control overeating and may also lower your cholesterol by about 5 percent in some people.

EATING HEALTHY FOR LIFE, MOST OF THE TIME

There is no need to follow a meal plan to lose weight, just eat healthy most of the time. Eat something you like, healthy or not once or twice a week. If you eat something high in fat or sugar, then go back to healthy eating again.

Eating your favorite regular food once or twice a week is fine. Example: you may eat pizza with your favorite high fat topping for one meal or as a snack, this does not meal that you will have all meals that are high or sweets for the entire day. You may eat your favorite candy bar at times, try eating half if you can. Just do not count calories or fat grams, it does not work.

You can lose weight without following a meal plan. You should follow a sensible and nutritious lower-fat, reduced sugar, eating pattern as much as possible with plenty of whole grains, fresh fruits, and vegetables. Fat calories are stored in the body more easily than that of protein or carbohydrate calories.

Overweight people consume a great deal of diet soda. The more diet soda they drink, the more they need to eat. Studies have shown that the brain has a conditioning response to the sweet taste. The brain associates the sweet taste with new energy entering the body. The sweet taste stimulates our taste buds. The brain signals the liver to prepare for the new incoming energy from the sweet taste of sugar. If the sweet taste is not followed by the nutrients, hunger sets in and there is a need to eat. The brain does not differentiate between the sweet taste from the sugar or aspartame, which is used to sweeten diet soda and other foods. If you do consume diet soda or drink a beverage that contains aspartame, other sweetener or sugar, drink it with your meals, not in between. It is necessary for you to follow Section A, read and learn Section A and follow it as much as possible. After a few weeks you will learn how easy it is to eat healthier most of the time. Do not be so concerned with weight loss. Be more concerned with not gaining any additional weight. When you eat healthy for life, it is a form of prevention for any health problems that may occur in the future or controlling any present medical conditions. Example: men in America suffer from more prostate problems than Asian men and this is due to a high fat intake. When Asian men come to America and if they start eating our diet which is high in fat, then the prostate cancer in these men also increase or surpass men in America.

Prevention is the key for keeping your body healthier for any condition, and the first step starts with the A, B, C, D, Ease of eating healthy for life. When you eat healthy and follow necessary measurements, you should have no problem in controlling and maintaining your weight throughout life.

During the time that you are reading and learning how to eat healthier, if you happen to go out on a special occasion such as a wedding, birthday party, etc., enjoy the special occasion and eat the food that is being served. That will be your one day to enjoy yourself and then start back eating healthier again soon after. If eating gooey for one day is going to cause a problem, then something is definitely wrong and I recommend you have a complete physical examination or speak to a medical doctor, professional nutritional practitioner, a therapist, or you may need the service of a weight loss coach. Weight loss coaching can be conducted over the phone.

YOU MUST EAT TO LOSE WEIGHT

You should be eating on an average of six times a day. Diets do not work. Eating will keep the metabolic rate up, and you will burn calories and fat by keeping the body working. Every time you starve yourself, your body's survival instinct will take over, and fights to preserve its fat stored. Your body becomes more able at keeping its fat with every low calorie diet you go on. When you come off the diet, and start eating again, you will probably gain all that weight you lost back and more. If you continue dieting, or starving yourself, your metabolism will slow down so much that small portions of food can make you gain weight. Without the proper amount of food throughout the day, your body has no reason to work harder. You must eat enough to keep your metabolic rate up. The best way to lose weight and keep it off is to eat more fat burning foods along with moderate exercise/physical activity, and you must also control your fat and sugar intake too.

LOW CALORIE DIETS AND LEAN MUSCLE TISSUE

Extremely fast weight loss caused by diets too low in calories will cause the breakdown of many lean muscle tissues. Low calorie dieting causes the body to "waste" to survive. The body requires certain levels of glucose in the blood. When the calories are too restricted, it will deprive the body of an adequate supply of glucose. The body must then breakdown tissue to raise the glucose back to a required level. This can only be done with the breakdown of lean muscle tissue and not fat. Fat cannot be converted to glucose, only to amino acids and protein. Starvation will result in the loss of lean tissue. With the loss of lean tissue, your calorie requirement will decrease; only lean tissue burns calories. When you begin eating again, your body will be less able to burn the same number of calories as before, because of less lean tissue. When you start back eating, the excess calories will be stored as fat and the weight will be regained. Depriving yourself of calories will make you depressed at times, mentally worthless, and eventually fatter. A diet too low in calories can also cause sleep disorders. You must eat regularly to stay alert and to prevent bingeing. Eating more often and consuming more higher fiber, lower fat, lower calorie foods will stabilize your insulin, maintain your energy levels, and help you lose fat and keep you from gaining weight.

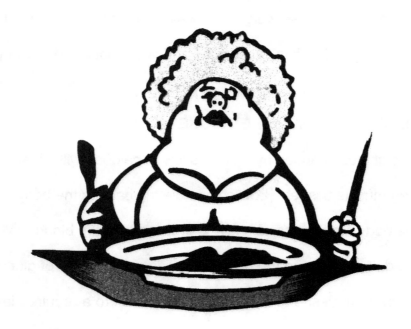

WHY EAT BREAKFAST

Eating breakfast will wake up your metabolism and start the body working. This will make you better able to burn fat throughout the day. Breakfast skippers usually end up eating more calories per day than people who eat breakfast. Eating breakfast, you will perform better at work and with other activities throughout the day. People who eat breakfast are usually slimmer than those who skip breakfast, and they usually eat less, and usually avoid eating more fatty foods.

PRE-BREAKFAST: FRESH FRUIT AND COLD WATER

Upon waking up in the morning before your daily shower, start out by drinking a tall glass of cold water. The cold from the water will cause your body temperature to drop down below normal. Your body must maintain itself at a normal body temperature of 98.6°. The chill will wake up your metabolism. As your metabolism starts to speed up, your body temperature will return back within normal range, and you will start burning calories and fat grams better throughout the day. After your morning shower, you can start eating your pre-breakfast (fruit only).

Avoid eating a heavy breakfast when you wake up in the morning. Your body is actually still using the food consumed the day before and will provide you with the required energy and you will be more alert and energetic. From the time you wake up in the morning until around 11 a.m. you should eat nothing but fresh fruit. You can eat as much fruit as you want during the morning, right up until about thirty minutes before you eat any other food.

You must remember that the traditional breakfast forces the body to work for hours using up needed energy to digest food. Food can spend from three hours or more in the stomach digesting. Energy cannot begin to be built up for other body activities until food is absorbed from the intestines.

After getting up in the morning or whatever time your day starts, eat nothing but fresh fruit. Eat as much as you want, but still train yourself not to overeat any food. Calories from fresh fruit is not a problem, only when fresh fruit is altered by heat, processed, or consumed together with other foods, negative things occur. If fresh fruit is consumed correctly and on an empty stomach, the high quality calories from the high water content in fresh fruit will not cause weight gain, but will provide the body with the needed energy to enhance weight loss and more calories and fat grams will be burned.

The food must be broken down and changed into glucose, fructose, glycerine, fatty acid, and amino acids. The brain can only function with glucose. More over, research study reported that sugar fructose enhanced weight loss. The study was conducted on fruit sugar fructose v. common sugar sucrose. The group that consumed their beverages sweetened with fruit sugar fructose ate about 470 calories less daily than those people who used common sugar sucrose as a sweetener. This is remarkable because the rule of thumb, it only takes about 500 calories less a day to lose a pound a week.

SKIPPING BREAKFAST IS NOT THE ANSWER

When it comes to eating healthy, not eating or skipping meals is the biggest mistake you can make. Many people feel that it is fine to not eat breakfast or even skip lunch or avoid snacking. What happens is that you become so hungry that you may start binge eating. You will eat anything in sight and it is usually the wrong kind of foods. When you skip meals and become extremely hungry, your body responds negatively and it believes that it is starving. If this type of eating pattern continues, fat will start to deposition in your stomach area, your backside, in your face, or elsewhere. This problem could be prevented by never skipping meals most of the time. The worst thing you can do for your metabolism is not eating. You need to eat five to six smaller meals throughout the course of a day. Eating small meals more frequently throughout the day your body will not perceive that it is starving. You will never get too hungry and this will help control binge eating. Small meals are easier to digest, and will speed up your metabolism, which will cause you to burn more calories and fat grams and your body will stay leaner. People who do not eat breakfast and many also skip lunch or avoid snacking throughout the day usually have more body fat.

THE POWER OF FRUIT – THE MOST IMPORTANT FOOD YOU CAN EAT IS FRUIT, AND IT WILL ALSO ENHANCE WEIGHT LOSS

I consider fruit the miracle food because of its many benefits. Fruit is the most important food and has the highest water content for cleansing the body and it leaves no toxic residue in the body and requires little or no energy for digestion. If fruit is properly consumed, it promotes good health, longer life, a more healthy looking body, provides needed energy for physical body functions and will enhance weight loss. Fruit is the only food that contains the five essentials of life and in the correct percentage. Fruit contains glucose for fuel, amino acids, minerals, vitamins and fatty acids. If fruits are properly chewed, eaten and properly consumed on an empty stomach, it will not stay in the stomach for long period of time. Fruit is pre-digested and does not need to digest in the stomach and requires little or no energy to be digested. Fruits pass quickly into the intestines and the nutrients are absorbed and used immediately. Food that contain a low-water content is more densed and will stay in the stomach from 1 ½ up to 4 hours of digesting. If foods are not consumed in the correct combination, it can stay in the stomach for 8 hours or more digesting before moving into the intestines. Digestion of food requires more energy than any other body functions.

All fruit only remain in the stomach for no more than twenty or thirty minutes with the exception of bananas, dates, and dried fruits which have less water contents and they will require more time to pass through the stomach, fifty minutes up to an hours. Fresh fruit is intended to pass quickly through the stomach if consumed properly. If fresh fruit or fresh fruit juice is consumed with other foods, it will stay in the stomach for a very long period of time together with the total meal. Shortly after fresh fruit or fruit juice come into contact with the other foods and in contact with the digestive juices in the stomach, the food will almost immediately start to rot. Most people believe that when fresh fruit is consumed right after a meal, that it will settle the stomach, this is not true. Eating fresh fruit before or right after the meal is the cause of most upset stomachs. It is also believed that eating fresh fruit before the meal will help prevent overeating. This is true, but you still need to let twenty to thirty minutes to pass before consuming anything after eating fruit to prevent the food from spoiling in the stomach and more time is necessary to pass after eating bananas, dates, or dried fruits.

The correct way to eat fruit is fresh. The body utilizes fruit best in its natural state. Fresh fruit must always be eaten on an empty stomach. As long as the stomach is empty, you can eat all the fresh fruit you want. Never eat anything right after you have eaten fresh fruit. After you have consumed any of the foods, do not eat fresh fruit for about three hours. After eating a meat meal, do not eat any fresh fruit for about four hours. If you eat a lot of junk foods or a lot of any other foods in different

combinations, do not eat any fresh fruit for about eight hours, or you may

just want to start back eating fresh fruit again the following day. Let's say

that you go out to eat at your favorite diner on a weekend day and you

treat yourself to an early morning traditional breakfast, look at what will

occur:

TRADITIONAL BREAKFAST ORDERED	FRESH FRUIT OR FRUIT JUICE EATEN WITH OTHER FOODS IN THE STOMACH
- Orange juice	The orange juice is usually pasteurized and made from concentrates which is pure acid. Pure acid will not aid weight loss.
- Toast or pancakes	The carbohydrates in the stomach ferments.
- Bacon and eggs	The protein in the stomach putrefies (rots).
- Bowl of fresh fruit said to settle the stomach	Fresh fruit is intended to pass quickly through the stomach into the intestine, but when consumed incorrectly, fresh fruit will stay in the stomach for hours along with the total traditional breakfast and spoil.

Because fruit has a high-water content of about 80 percent or more

cleaning life giving water, fruit will help remove toxic waste from the body

and help prevent waste build-up. It is necessary for the body to be

constantly cleaned of toxic waste. The best way to remove unwanted

30

toxic waste and to prevent toxic waste from building up in the body is by eating more foods with a high-water content in the correct combination. Fresh fruit has the highest water content of any food. It is the perfect, most nutritious food that is most beneficial to sustain life and also will enhance weight loss too.

ACID – ALKALINE BALANCE, FRUIT AND WEIGHT CONTROL

Acid – Alkaline balance is extremely important to normal physiology. Body fluids are maintained at a PH ranging between 7.35 and 7.45 which is slightly alkaline. Extended PH imbalances of any kind are not well tolerated by the body. It is believed by some that high acidity may deplete bones because the body has to take alkalizing minerals (especially calcium) from bones to keep the blood from dropping into the acid range. A PH below 7 indicates acid, a PH above 7 indicates alkalinity. A PH of 7.0 measures exact neutrality. Alkalinity can be increased by eating more fruits and vegetables. Many believe most fruit will increase the acid in the blood. Citrus fruits like lemons, oranges, grapefruits, pineapples, and peaches contain organic acids. These acids are weak and they do not increase the acidity of the stomach. All fruits become alkaline once they go into the stomach if properly consumed. The organic acids in fruits are oxidized to yield energy, carbon dioxide and water. Acid producing flesh foods like meat, poultry and fish consumption should be controlled. Alkalinity can be increased by consuming less meat and sweets and eating more fruits and vegetables. We consume too much flesh foods in this country. It is necessary to maintain a proper acid-alkaline balance in the body. Try to eat no more than 6 oz. of flesh protein in a day. If large amounts of meat are eaten in a day, an extremely large amount of energy will be used up for digestion and not enough energy will be left over for other body activities like weight control. People who eat less meat for long period of time, for years have no protein deficiencies because of other non-flesh foods like fruits, vegetables, beans and all nuts and seeds. Eating meat is fine on a healthy meal plan for life, but it is necessary to control your portion size.

HYDRATE WITH COLD WATER FOR WEIGHT LOSS

I recommend that you drink a tall ice cold glass of water just before or with each meal. This will ensure that you get your needed amount of daily water for proper body hydration. We need water for all our bodily processes which include digestion of food, elimination of waste, circulation, and breathing. Proper hydration will aid your body muscles in using carb correctly and you will burn more fat. The more ice cold water you drink, the more calories you will burn. If you drink an eight glass of ice cold water as compared to water at room temperature, you can burn an additional 9.25 calories or more. The recommended water daily for proper hydration is eight 8 oz. glasses a day.

WATER AND WEIGHT LOSS

Water is a nutrient and it is the most important one. Water is also the most abundant substance in the body. All the body tissues contain some amount of water. Our body weight is made up of 10 to 12 gallons of water. During the daily function of the body there is about 10 or more cups of water loss. (perspiration, eliminating and it is also needed for the process of breathing.)

Water is also needed as follows:

- for elimination

- to transport nutrients throughout the body

- to transport oxygen

- to provide protection and cushion for vital organs of the body

- provides.lubrication for the joint

- waste products and internal secretion

- regulates body temperature

WATER NEEDED DAILY

2 quarts or more is best for the normal individual each day, but try to drink no less than 6 to 8 cups daily.

DRINKING COLD MILK OR WATER AND WEIGHT CONTROL

After waking up in the morning, you should have a pre-breakfast, before you shower or bathe, drink a glass of ice-cold low fat milk or a tall glass of ice water. The coldness from the cold water or milk will cause the body temperature to drop. This in return will cause your metabolism to wake up. The body temperature will need to return back to normal and you will start to burn calories. This is like getting your body's motor a jumpstart and anything you eat through the day will burn off easier. Everyone cannot drink milk, but if you can, the protein in the milk will also help energize the brain. Also, drinking water just before you eat will help fill you up faster and may prevent overeating.

WATER VERSUS HUNGER

At times we may feel a need to eat thinking that hunger has set in. You should first try to drink a tall glass of water. You may find out that you are only thirsty, which may prevent overeating and help suppress the appetite. If you are still hungry after you drink some water, have a healthy snack.

ABNORMAL WATER RETENTION – (THIS IS RARE)

Drinking excessive amounts of water may accumulate in your tissues, which may be the cause of your weight problems. Large amount of water weighs more than fat. You should always consult your doctor before starting any weight loss program. He or she can tell if there are any other problems other than weight.

MEAL SCHEDULE

(Use this as a guide)

Pre-breakfast	7 a.m. to 10:30 a.m. (Upon waking up, fresh fruit, fresh fruit juice, and cold water).
Breakfast, light	11 a.m.
Lunch	1 p.m.
Snack	3 p.m.
Dinner	6 p.m.
Bedtime, small snack as needed	8 p.m.

If you do not eat for example regular breakfast, lunch, or snacks, try making bag meals. It may be convenient for you because of your schedule to pre-prep and carry some meals or combine bag meals. Try to eat at least two healthy smaller portions solid meals a day. You need to eat five to six smaller meals a day to keep your metabolism rated. You will continue to burn calories and fat grams better throughout the day. Remember you need to eat to lose weight. It does not take will power to lose weight, but just a little knowledge. You need to start out by shopping right and learn to eat healthier most of the time.

BREAKFAST

(Select One Choice or Use This List As A Guide)

Allow twenty to thirty minutes to pass before eating breakfast after having your pre-breakfast of only fresh fruit and cold water. If you have a banana, dates or dried fruit, let forty five minutes up to one hour to pass before eating breakfast or any meal. With each meal drink a tall glass of ice water or iced tea sweetened with Splenda. Use wheat bread if you can.

1. 2 slices of toast (wheat or white)
    1 slice American cheese
    *For hot cheese sandwich, place cheese between hot toast right away.

2. 1 toasted bagel (wheat or white)
    1 tablespoon peanut butter

3. 1 hard boiled egg
    1 small roll with fruit spread

4. 1 toasted bagel (wheat or white)
    1 tablespoon cottage cheese spread

5. 1 bowl 40% bran flakes
    1 glass of 1% milk or skim milk

6. 2 pancakes topped with ½ cup unsweetened apples sauce (not diet)

7. 1 toasted English muffin (wheat or white)
    1 tablespoon peanut butter with fruit spread

8. 1 to 1 ½ bowl of hot cooked Farina with 1% milk or skim milk

9. 1 bowl all bran with 1% milk or skim milk

10. 2 toasted waffles topped with ½ cup plain vanilla yogurt, reduced fat

BREAKFAST

11. 1 bagel cheese melt
(First toast bagel, then place 1 oz. slice of American cheese between bagel, let melt and serve.)

12. Potatoes and eggs
1 medium diced, peeled potato, steamed or boiled
2 egg whites, 1 egg yolk, 1 teaspoon cold water
season to taste and mix.

    First slightly boil the diced potatoes until firm, discard water. Then, saute the potatoes until slightly brown in nonstick skillet in Smart Balance buttery spread or coat skillet with olive oil. When potatoes are done, add egg mixture.

13. French toast (wheat or white)
2 slices of bread topped with ½ cup unsweetened applesauce (not diet) or stewed apples with Splenda seasoned with cinnamon or served with fruit spread.

    *egg mixture for French toast
2 egg whites, 1 egg yolk, 1% or skim milk, vanilla flavoring, cinnamon, and nutmeg. Blend all ingredients together. Dip bread into mixture. Pan fry in nonstick skillet in Smart Balance buttery spread.

14. Bacon, lettuce and tomato sandwich
2 slices of toast (wheat or white)
2 slices of tomatoes with lettuce
1 slice of Canadian bacon steamed
(Serve 1 ounce of cooked bacon).

15. 2 slices whole wheat toast with fruit spread
1 hard boiled egg

16. 1 to 1 ½ cup cooked oatmeal, sweetened with Splenda and sprinkled with 1 teaspoon of chopped nuts and cinnamon (No milk).

17. 1 bowl Shredded Wheat with 1% milk or skim milk

BREAKFAST

18.   Scrambled egg sandwich on roll
1 toasted hard roll
2 egg whites, 1 slice low fat cheese (1 gram of fat or less)
*White of the eggs plus 1 teaspoon of water, season to taste and mix. Then add diced cheese. Scramble mixture in nonstick skillet in Smart Balance buttery spread. You may use egg substitutes in place of fresh eggs.

19.   Grits topped with scrambled eggs
1 cup of cooked quick grits (follow package directions).
2 egg whites, 1 egg yolk, 1 teaspoon water, season to taste and mix. Scramble and cook in nonstick skillet in Smart Balance buttery spread.

20.   Chipped beef and toast (wheat or white)
For chipped beef with gravy (white sauce),
*Follow the cooking directions on jar, but substitute skim milk and Smart Balance buttery spread for regular butter.
Chipped beef mixture can be served over 1 or 2 slices of plain toast or 1 medium low-fat biscuit made from reduced fat Bisquick mix.

21.   Ham and egg sandwich
1 toasted English muffin
1 ounce slice of cooked turkey ham
¼ cup egg substitute, plain or with thin slices of green bell pepper and fresh sliced onions
*Saute egg substitute use nonstick skillet in Smart Balance buttery spread. If green peppers and fresh onion are added, they are to be sauted first, then add egg substitute, season to taste.

22.   Toasted English muffin and peanut butter
1 English muffin
2 teaspoons peanut butter (smooth)
*You can also add peanut butter topped with a little fruit spread.

You do not have to give up treats to eat healthy. On one day of the week, treat yourself if you like.

23.   Americans love sausage, egg and toast breakfast
2 slices of toast with fruit spread
2 links cooked sausage, 1 oz each with 1 gram of fat or less per ounce – very lean meat
1 egg cooked in Smart Balance buttery spread

BREAKFAST

24.   Americans love bacon, egg and hot biscuit breakfast
1 hot biscuit with Smart Balance buttery spread
2 slices bacon, regular and very lean
1 egg cooked in Smart Balance buttery spread
*Cook bacon under broiler or grill on a rack to allow fat to drip off.
Do not fry.
*Cook lean bacon in microwave to reduce fat.
*For biscuits, follow directions on package of reduced fat Bisquick.

LUNCH OR DINNER

HELPFUL TIPS TO PREVENT OVEREATING (PRE-MEAL)

Have a light appetizer, pre-meal, or small snack before eating your main meal. This may help prevent overeating. You may want to have a light soup or broth and a healthy salad with a glass of ice cold water or unsweetened beverage just before you eat your main meal. You may eat 20% less fat and calories because the pre-meal or appetizer will make your stomach fuller, cut the hunger, and should help prevent overeating.

PRE-MEAL JUST BEFORE EATING YOUR MAIN MEAL

(Use this as a guide)

- Toss green salad with reduced fat or fat-free dressing
- 1 glass cold ice water
- 1 glass of unsweetened iced tea or sweetened with Splenda
- 1 glass of cold club soda or tonic water
- 1 cup of unsweetened jello
- 1 large bowl of broth, 98% fat free
- 1 glass watered cold tomato juice seasoned to taste
- 1 cup watered down hot canned tomato or other soup
- 1 cup watered down cream of chicken or other healthy cream soup. use Campbell's Healthy Request, 30% less sodium, 98% fat free.

*The quick 2 easy directions
1 can of water added to
1 can of cream soup
½ cup per serving

My easy recipe changed to:
2 cans of water added to
1 can of cream soup, onion powder, garlic powder and pepper to taste. 1 cup per serving. This will help fill you up and you will have more soup to sip one and still save calories and fat grams. You may try to dilute the soup ½ to 1 cup more water and season to taste. You will have a lighter soup, save on calories and fat grams.

*Diluted soup or fat-free broth can also be consumed between meals as a snack to help control hunger. At times you may not be too hungry, but just want to eat something light and not a full main meal. You can have a healthy cup of soup with a ½ sandwich or a few snack crackers, or with a light salad.

Remember, do not use fresh fruit or fruit juice as an appetizer or pre-meal to prevent overeating. Unless you can time the consumption of fruit right avoid same. Fresh fruit should be eaten on an empty stomach. If three hours has passed after eating your last meal, you can have a piece of fresh fruit, but not less than twenty minutes before the meal or no less than forty five minutes before a meal if you eat a banana, dates or dried fruit. Let's say that you are cooking your lunch or dinner meal and you know that you did not eat anything for the past 3 hours. Since you are eating smaller, lighter meals now, 3 hours should be enough time to allow the previous meal to digest and travel out of the stomach. A piece of fresh fruit or fruit juice would be a nice treat. This will control your hunger and prevent overeating.

DESSERT AS A SNACK OR PRE-MEAL

Lower calorie desserts can also be used as a snack or pre-meal. It is not necessary to have a dessert after the main meal. The dessert can be eaten between meals as one of your daily snacks to help control hunger and to prevent overeating. Some say by eating the dessert before a meal will also control overeating. For example: eat 2 each ginger snaps with a cup of hot tea or a few reduced fat snack crackers followed by the lunch or supper meal may help control the portion size for the overeater.

To help prevent overeating instead of soup or salad at times you may want to have a light snack or dessert before the meal, use this list as a guide:

- 1 cup sugar free jello with 1 teaspoon fat free or reduced fat sour cream

- 1 cup regular jello

- ½ cup jello with cool whip, fat-free topping

- ½ cup instant pudding, made with skim milk

- 1 cup whipped cold skim milk flavored with vanilla extract and sweetened with Splenda

- ½ cup fat free, sugar free frozen yogurt

- cup water fruit ice

- 2 ginger snap cookies with ½ cup cold skim milk

- 1 cup popcorn, low fat

- 1 pc. rice cake with hot tea

- ¼ cup salsa with celery dipper

- Celery sticks stuffed with 1 tablespoon of smooth cream cheese filling, fat free, reduced fat

- Hot cocoa, 1 tablespoon unsweetened cocoa powder added to 1 cup hot water, sweetened with Splenda, plus 1 tablespoon non dairy liquid

- Dill pickle, large

- 5 reduced fat snack crackers with cup of hot tea

LUNCH
(Select One Choice or Use This List As A Guide)

1. Cup of 98% fat free broth
   ½ cup tuna
   5 saltine crackers
   toss green salad

2. Cup of hot canned low fat vegetable soup thin out with water and seasoned to taste
   1 hard boiled egg
   1 medium baked sweet potato
   lettuce and tomato salad

3. Large glass of chilled tomato juice ½ water, ½ juice seasoned to taste
   turkey on small roll
   2 thin sliced turkey with thin slices of cucumber and tomato
   *May use large roll, but remove some of the bread inside.

4. Large glass of iced tea
   Large bowl of hot fat free chicken broth 98% fat free
   Noodles and cheese
   1 cup of hot cooked noodles, mix in
   ½ cup of cottage cheese, add pepper, toss and serve

5. Cup of any canned low fat cream soup diluted with water season to taste.
   Pita bread sandwich with balsamic dressing
   1 oz. diced cooked chicken breast
   chopped lettuce
   diced tomatoes
   diced cucumbers
   Mix dry ingredients and place in pita bread, salt and pepper with Balsamic Vinegar and sprinkle inside pita bread

6. Low fat broth
   Stir fried chicken and rice combination dish
   This can be easy to make from left over chicken and rice.
   1 oz. cooked lean diced chicken breast
   ¾ cup cooked brown or white rice
   Toss all together and stir fry with cooking spray with diced green pepper, diced onion, sliced fresh or canned mushroom and season to taste.

LUNCH

7. Large glass of chilled tomato juice ½ water, ½ juice season to taste
    Hard egg and bean salad
    1 cup of chilled canned green beans with diced tomatoes
    diced onions, vinegar, mustard, season to taste, toss and serve
    garnish with 1 sliced or diced hard boiled egg with low fat or fat free
    dressing

8. Cup of low fat soup ½ water, ½ soup, season to taste or
    Large glass of iced tea sweetened with Splenda
    1 pita bread egg salad sandwich (wheat or white)
    boiled egg (2 white, 1 egg yolk) mix with 1 teaspoon mayonnaise
    and 1 teaspoon of mustard) season to taste.
    Side order of sliced cucumber
    sliced tomatoes and pickles, if desired.

9. Cup of fat free broth or 98% fat free
    Large glass of iced tea sweetened with Splenda
    1 baked chicken breast
    1 baked sweet potato
    slightly cooked broccoli top with tomato salsa

10. Cup cream of potato soup 98% fat free diluted with water or fat free
    broth 98% fat free
    Large glass of cold club soda
    4 pcs. sardines
    6 saltine crackers
    vegetable platter – tomatoes, cucumbers, celery, carrots, and low
    fat homemade dip or any reduced fat salad dressing

11. Large cup of low fat broth 98% fat free
    Large glass of unsweetened cold gingerale

    Stuffed Tomatoes
    Large tomato cut almost ¼"
    ½ cup tuna with diced celery and onion if desired
    1 tablespoon of mayonnaise and 1 tablespoon of mustard mix and
    place into tomato served on lettuce bed
    Glass of iced tea sweetened with Splenda

12. Grill fish on a bed of canned vegetable
    2 oz of fresh or frozen cod, flounder, haddock or halibut
    1 cup toss succotash and fresh tomato together with a little
    Balsamic Vinegar, season to taste, onion and bell pepper if desired.

LUNCH

13. Cup of hot diluted tomato soup, seasoned
Turkey sausage/pita bread or Italian bread
1 boiled or grilled low fat Italian sausage
Grilled green peppers and onion topping or
red onion with red sauce or sauerkraut or both

14. Cup of low fat cream of chicken ½ diluted with water

Grilled garden vegetable hero sandwich
Zucchini thinly sliced
Red pepper thin sliced
Eggplant thinly sliced
Mushrooms thinly sliced
Olive oil
Season vegetable to taste, sprinkle with olive oil, let marinate.
Grill vegetable or cook under broiler, until firm

15. Large bowl of hot low fat beef broth, or fat free
Large glass of cold iced tea sweetened with Splenda
turkey sandwich with mustard
2 thin slices of white turkey 1 ½ oz.
2 slices of thin toast or pita bread
lettuce and tomato
Spread with mustard or sprinkle with a low fat or fat free dressing

DINNER

(Select One Choice or Use This List As A Guide)

1. 4 ounces lean sirloin or flank steak, seasoned and grilled. Example: spread prepared mustard over steak, then grill in oven, turn steak, spread with mustard, complete cooking, and serve.
1 cup cooked string beans
½ cup beets

2. 4 ounces grilled salmon with lemon or grilled with low sodium soy sauce
1 cup cooked broccoli
½ cup cooked whole kernel corn

3. 6 ounces cooked steamed shrimp or sauted with Smart Balance buttery spread in nonstick skillet
1 cup steam cabbage
½ cup stir fry bell green pepper and mushrooms
*You may mix shrimp, bell pepper and mushrooms together (stir-fry)

4. 4 ounces of chicken fillet (without skin), seasoned and grilled (mustard, low sodium soy sauce, or Worchester sauce)
1 cup cooked carrots
½ cup beets

5. 4 ounces cooked fish fillet (use fresh or frozen fish) seasoned to taste (baked, grilled, or broiled)
1 ½ cups broccoli and cauliflower

6. 8 medium sardines with mustard (canned)
1 cup cooked spinach
½ cup cooked carrots

7. 4 ounces turkey burger (salt, pepper, onion and garlic powder) or season to taste, and grill
1 to 1 ½ cups California vegetables or mixed vegetables

8. 4 ounces lean veal chop, trim off the fat, baked, broiled, or grilled seasoned to taste with mustard, low sodium soy sauce or Worchester sauce, if desired
1 to 1 ½ cups sliced carrots and peas

DINNER

9.   4 ounces sliced turkey breast or grilled turkey fillet
     (buy in supermarket, pre-packaged), season to taste with mustard,
     low sodium soy sauce, etc.
     1 cup brussel sprouts
     ½ cup baby carrots

10. 4 ounces cooked chicken fillet (without the skin) seasoned if
     desired with (a) mustard (b) low sodium soy sauce or
     Worcestershire sauce, grilled, baked, or broiled
     1 cup steamed cabbage
     acorn or butternut baked with Smart Balance and sprinkle with salt,
     pepper and Splenda (sweetener) and bake

11. 4 ounces of grilled salmon
     1 cup cooked green beans
     ½ cup mushrooms
     *You may mix vegetable together, season to taste and saute

12. 4 ounces chicken fillet (without the skin) seasoned to taste,
     grilled with sweet and sour sauce or mustard
     1 cup turnip green, or spinach or other greens
     ½ cup carrots
     *Add Smart Balance to carrots and Splenda

13. 2 boiled frankfurters
     1 cup broccoli
     ½ cup corn

14. 4 ounces lean grilled pork chop grilled, baked or pan fried
     (Do not deep fry).
     1 cup asparagus
     ½ cup corn

15. 4 ounces of roast veal cutlet
     1 cup sliced yellow squash
     ½ cup green peas

SEASONING OF FOODS

You do not need to sacrifice taste or flavor when eating healthy for life. There are substitutes, replacements or alternatives on the market. If you have any health problems, always consult with your physician as needed. The following alternatives are my recommendations:

- Splenda – sugar replacement

- Smart Balance – butter or margarine replacement

- Cardia – salt alternative

SPLENDA

In place of sugar, it is a no calorie sweetener. Measure spoon for spoon like sugar and it can also be used for cooking and baking. It can be used by people who are diabetic and it is parve.

SMART BALANCE

Use it in place of butter or margarine as a buttery spread, as a seasoning, and for cooking and baking. It tastes like butter and contains 50% or more less fat and calories. It has no hydrogenated oils, is trans-fatty acid free, is lactose free, is parve and it is said to improve the cholesterol.

CARDIA

This salt alternative has 54% less sodium than table salt. It was formulated for hypertensive patients who have a difficult time reducing their salt (sodium) intake by following a control diet. It can be used as a seasoning or in cooking. It is recommended that if you have a medical problem, consult with your physician first.

EATING HEALTHY FOR LIFE, MOST OF THE TIME

There is no need to follow a meal plan to lose weight; just eat healthy most of the time. Eat something you like, healthy or not once or twice a week. When you eat something high in fat or sugar, you should go back to healthy eating again.

Eating your favorite regular food once or twice a week is fine. Example: you may eat a pizza with your favorite high fat topping for one meal or as a snack, this does not mean that you will have all meals that are high in fat or sweets for the entire day. You may eat your favorite candy bar at times, try eating half if you can. Just do not count calories or fat grams. It does not work.

You can lose weight without following a meal plan. You should follow a sensible and nutritious lower-fat eating pattern as much as possible with plenty of whole grains, fresh fruits, and vegetables. Fat calories are stored in the body more readily than that of protein or carbohydrate calories. Do not drink diet soda or eat any diet foods that contain aspartame (Nutra-Sweet) or other substitutes.

Overweight people consume a great deal of diet soda. The more diet soda they drink, the more they need to eat. Studies have shown that the brain has a conditioning response to the sweet taste. The brain associates the sweet taste with new energy entering the body. The sweet taste stimulates our taste buds. The brain signals the liver to prepare for the new incoming energy from the sweet taste of sugar. If the sweet taste is not followed by the nutrients, hunger sets in and there is a need to eat. The brain does not differentiate between the sweet taste from the sugar or aspartame, which is used to sweeten diet soda and other foods.

Note:

1.   Eat in moderation. You are not provided with a meal regimen, but you are provided with a list of foods to eat and avoid. Use this list as a guide.

2.   Eat more lean, lower-fat beef, poultry, and white meat turkey with no skin and eat more fish.

3.   Try to limit meat to 6 ounces per day.

4.   Drink ice-cold water before each meal. Drink plenty of cold water throughout the day.

5.   Select foods that are higher in fiber, whole grain bread and cereal and fresh fruits and vegetables. Eat more complex carbohydrates. Avoid refined carbohydrates or concentrated sweets. Select foods with high fiber content.

EATING FIVE OR SIX TIMES A DAY IS BETTER

You will most likely eat what is stocked in the house. Eat more often, eat less, but shop healthy.

1.   Breakfast

2.   Snack

3.   Lunch

4.   Snack

5.   Dinner

6.   Snack

YOU WILL NEVER GET HUNGRY

Starting out by eating a healthy breakfast and you will burn food better in the morning and will wake up your metabolism. Continue to eat smaller meals within closer intervals. It will keep your metabolism raised and in return you should burn more calories and fat and you will never go hungry.

This guide is to be used for weight loss and weight maintenance. Avoid higher fat foods as much as possible and foods high in sugar.

You are not provided with a meal regimen, but are provided with a list of foods allowed and foods to avoid. Cut the fat, reduce sugar. Use this guide to increase your knowledge for A B C D – Ease for healthy eating, weight-loss and maintenance. Eating healthy is easy. There is no need to follow a meal plan.

FOOD	FOOD ALLOWED	FOOD RESTRICTED OR CUT BACK AS MUCH AS POSSIBLE
Poultry	• Cooking method: baked, boiled, broiled, pan broiled, roasted, stewed, poached, simmered, grilled, stir frying, braising, trim visible fat. • Buying poultry- very lean: Eat more white meat chicken, turkey, and Cornish hen with no skin. • Lean meat poultry: dark meat chicken and turkey with no skin. • Ground chicken and turkey: when possible have meat market ground fresh white meat only. May buy ground turkey or chicken prepackaged. Must be very lean – read package.	Avoid fried meats or poultry. Do not add flour, cornstarch, or puree to sauces or stew before fat is removed (defat).
Wild Game	• Buying wild game – very lean meat: Duck or pheasant with no skin, venison, buffalo, ostrich. • Lean meat wild game: Goose with no skin, rabbit, and squirrel.	Avoid high fat duck or pheasant with skin and high fat goose with skin. Also avoid domestic duck or goose, if eaten, drain off fat well.

FOOD	FOOD ALLOWED	FOOD RESTRICTED OR CUT BACK AS MUCH AS POSSIBLE
Beef	• There are 3 types or grade of beef: select, choice, and prime. • Buy select or choice grade of beef. Choice grades or cuts of beef are the leanest. Select cuts of beef are only slightly leaner than choice cuts. Markets may not carry the select cuts, so it is okay to buy the choice cuts of beef. • Lean steaks and roast select or choice (sirloin, top loin, flank, tender loin, T-bone, porter house, beef cubes, eye rounds, top round, round tip, bottom round, chuck, rump, chopped beef – lean only.	Avoid or buy less prime grades or cuts of beef. Prime beef has more fat per ounce and also has more calories. Avoid fried meat, fatty meats, spiced or pickled meats, corned beef, canned meat, short ribs, and prime ribs. Avoid regular ground beef.
Pork	• Buying pork – lean meat: trim off fats. Lean pork chops and roasts pork tenderloin, sirloin, center loin, top loin, pork leg, shank, rump, fresh ham, Canadian bacon. Sausage with 1 gram or less fat per ounce – read labels.	Avoid fried pork, spareribs, ground pork, pork sausages (bratwurst), Italian, knockwurst, Polish smoked sausage, patty or link, ham hocks, pigs feet, pork cutlets, scrapples, pork butt, canned pork, salted pork, chitterlings, bacons.
Lamb	• Buying lamb: roast, chop, leg – trim off fat.	Avoid rib roast, ground lamb.
Veal	• Buying veal: lean chop or roast.	Avoid veal cutlets, ground veal.
Processed Meat	• Buying processed meat: lean meat – processed sandwich meat with 1 gram or less of fat per ounce.	Avoid high fat processed sandwich meats with 8 grams or less fat per ounce (bologna, pimento loaf, and salami).
Other Meats: Hotdogs	• Buying hotdogs: 1 gram or less of fat per ounce – read package.	Avoid high fat hotdogs – 8 grams or less per ounce. Turkey, chicken, beef or pork franks.
Kidneys	• Buying kidneys – very lean meat.	**PLEASE NOTE:** Avoid kidney (high in cholesterol). If there is a cholesterol problem – eat rarely.

FOOD	FOOD ALLOWED	FOOD RESTRICTED OR CUT BACK AS MUCH AS POSSIBLE
Fish	• Buying fish: all fresh and frozen fish, salmon (fresh or canned), sardines (canned), herring (uncreamed), oyster, fresh or canned with no oil. • Any fish is good. • Fresh or frozen cod, flounder, haddock, halibut, trout, tuna, fresh or canned in water. Very lean shellfish – clams, crab, lobster, scallops, shrimp, and imitation shellfish.	Avoid fried fish, fish canned in oil and creamed herring.
Eggs	• Eat eggs three times a week. Egg whites as desired; cholesterol free egg substitute such as Eggbeaters.	Avoid cream or au gratin-for these recipes, use skim milk or lower fat cheeses.
Cheese	• Buying cheese: Non-fat or low-fat cottage cheese, grated parmesan, cheese made with skim milk such as ricotta, mozzarella, American cheese, Swiss, Monterey. • Look for other low-fat cheese on the market. Low calories cheeses – read the package. Very low fat cheeses – 1 gram or less of fat per ounce. Low-fat cheese – 3 grams or less of fat per ounce.	Avoid all regular cheese such as American cheese, blue cheese, cheddar cheese, Monterey, Swiss, ricotta, mozzarella. Medium fat cheese – 5 grams or less fat per ounce. Eat occasionally – feta, mozzarella and ricotta. Look for lower fat versions.
Dry Beans	• Beans and peas cooked: Adzuki beans, black beans, black-eye peas (cowpeas), chickpeas (garbanzo beans), cranberry beans, fava beans, great northern beans, green peas, lentils, lima beans, mung beans, navy beans, pigeon peas, pink beans, pinto beans, soybeans, split peas, white beans, yellow beans, red kidney beans.	Avoid cooking beans with butter, bacon, salt port, or any fatty meat. Avoid cooking beans with coconut and also avoid refried beans.

FOOD	FOOD ALLOWED	FOOD RESTRICTED OR CUT BACK AS MUCH AS POSSIBLE
Bread, Potatoes, Beans, etc.	• All enriched or whole grain bread or yeast rolls, bread sticks, graham crackers, melba toast, pretzels, matzos, rye wafers, saltines, unbuttered popcorn, pancakes, low-fat waffles, corn bread, oyster crackers, whole wheat crackers, rye crisp, white French, Italian bread, whole wheat bread, bagel, bread stocks, low-fat croutons, English muffins, frankfurter and hamburger buns, raisin bread, plain roll, rye bread, pumpernickel, tortilla. • Potatoes or substitute: macaroni, noodles, white or brown rice, spaghetti, sweet potato, yam, white potato, prepared white potato with no added fat, beans, peas, lentils, corn, lima beans, plantains, squash, acorn, butter nuts, cassava (yucca), taro root.	Avoid quick breads, muffins, biscuits, pancakes, doughnuts, fritters, crackling corn bread, fried corn bread, sweet rolls, hot bread unless made with very little fat, popcorn with butter, wheat germ, French fries, snacks – potato chips, corn chips, any bread with extra fat added. Avoid fried potatoes, chips, cream sauces made with whole milk, cheese sauces (cook without fat or oil).
Cereal	• Special K, Puffed Rice, rice cereal, Bran Flakes, All-Bran, Corn Flakes, bulgur cooked, grits cooked, corn-meal, Grape Nuts, wheat germ, Shredded Wheat, oatmeal, high fiber oatmeal, Wheatena, Farina, Super Bran, high fiber couscous, buckwheat, kasha, millets, mueslik, granola low fat.	Avoid cereals with coconut or nuts, any cereal with extra fat added, natural cereals. Avoid cereals with added sugar or frosted.

FOOD	FOOD ALLOWED	FOOD RESTRICTED OR CUT BACK AS MUCH AS POSSIBLE
Vegetables	• Fresh vegetables or frozen vegetables: asparagus, artichoke, bean sprouts, beets, Brussels sprouts, broccoli, cabbage (cooked), carrots, cauliflower (cooked), eggplant, celery (cooked), green peppers. • Green leafy vegetables: beets, chard, collards, dandelion, kale, mustard, spinach, turnips, kohlrabi, leek, mushrooms (cooked), no added fat salad, okra, onions, pea pods, rutabaga, string beans, turnips, summer squash, vegetable juice, sauerkraut, zucchini (cooked), tomatoes, water chestnuts, tomato juice. • These vegetables are good for salads and good with the main meal to help fill you up. they are also good to eat as a snack to prevent hunger, and may be used as desired: alfalfa sprouts, cucumbers, hot peppers, broccoli, endive, leeks, cauliflower, escarole, radishes, celery, lettuce, rhubarb, chicory, romaine, watercress, carrots, green peppers, tomato. • Seasonings can be very helpful in making vegetables taste better that will save on calories.	Avoid vegetables cooked with fatty meat, or additional fats, or butter, sour cream, do not add calories. Homemade low-fat sour cream is OK. Avoid commercially frozen vegetables, casserole with sauces, au gratin, creamed, or fried vegetables. Avocado and olives contain good fat, eat in moderation. Do not have commercially prepared salads with sour cream, regular mayonnaise, miracle whip, etc.

FOOD	FOOD ALLOWED	FOOD RESTRICTED OR CUT BACK AS MUCH AS POSSIBLE
Fruit	• All canned fruits unsweetened or in natural juice, dried fruit without sugar. Fruit juice – unsweetened or natural – apple, apple cider, cranberry, grapefruit, orange, pineapple, and prune. • Fresh fruit – apple, apricot, banana, blackberries, blueberries, cantaloupe, cherries, dates, grapefruit, grapes, honeydew, kiwi, mango, nectarine, orange, papaya, peach, pear, persimmon, plum, pineapple, pomegranate, raspberries, strawberries, tangerine, and watermelon. • Dried fruit – apples, apricots, dates, figs, pineapples, prunes, and raisins.	Avoid fruit nectar, fruit drinks with added sugar. Avocado is a good fruit but has fat and must be eaten only occasionally. Avoid dried fruits with sugar added.
Dessert	• All fruit, fruit whip, fruit pudding, gelatin, dessert made with egg white or gelatin, angel food cake, fruit ice, sherbet, plain pudding made with skim milk or egg whites, meringues, fig bars, ginger snaps, vanilla wafers, low-fat cookies, fruit spread, low-fat yogurt with cut fresh fruit or plain low-fat with or without fruit, fat-free yogurt, graham crackers, animal crackers, granola bars (fat-free), pumpkin made with skim milk or 1% milk yogurt, low-fat ice cream, and sorbet.	Avoid desserts made with whole milk, cream, butter, lard, coconut, chocolate, rich cookies, cakes, pastries, pie, and ice cream, high sugar desserts.
Fat – do not overeat any fat!	• Mono-unsaturated fat, poly-unsaturated fat, good health benefits in small amounts oils – canola, olive, peanut, corn, safflower, soybean, reduced fat salad dressing, nuts, olives, reduced fat mayonnaise, reduced fat miracle whip. If regular mayonnaise or miracle whip is used, use less. • Trans-fatty acid free butter, whipped butter.	Saturated – bacon, bacon fat, fat back, ham fat, lard, salt pork, shortening, gravy, coconut cream, half and half, regular cream cheese, regular sour cream, chitterlings, regular butter, margarine

HELPFUL TIPS FOR THE BUSY PERSON ON THE GO:

THE SURE WAY TO EAT BREAKFAST (PREPARE THE NIGHT BEFORE) –

BAG BREAKFAST FOR THE BUSY PERSON

- **CHEESE SANDWICH:** 2 slices whole wheat bread, 1 slice (1 ounce) reduced fat cheese

- **PEANUT BUTTER SANDWICH:** 2 slices raisin bread, 1 tablespoon reduced fat peanut butter, 1 cup diced melon in zipper lock bag

- **EGG SANDWICH:** 2 slices rye bread, 1 hard cooked egg sliced, 1 fresh orange or tangerine

HELPFUL TIPS TO PREVENT OVEREATING (PRE-MEAL)

Have a light appetizer, pre-meal, or small snack before eating your main meal. This may help prevent over-eating. You may want to have a light soup broth and a healthy salad with a glass of ice-cold water just before you eat your main meal. You may eat 20% less fat and calories because the pre-meal or appetizer will make your stomach fuller, cut the hunger, and help prevent over-eating.

- **PRE-MEAL:** 1 glass cold ice water or flavored lemon water - drink

- **PRE-MEAL:** 1 cup fat free chicken broth or 1 cup watered down hot tomato soup

- **PRE-MEAL:** Toss green salad with reduced fat or fat-free dressing

- **MAIN MEAL:** 4 ounces very lean steak with onion, ½ cup herb mashed potatoes and 1 cup steamed cabbage.

- ☐ **FROZEN DINNER REPLACEMENT:** To prevent constant meal prep, use frozen dinners at times. They are good and are more time saving. They are helpful for weight loss and maintenance. Choose a low fat frozen dinner that contains less than 10 grams of fat for the full meal or an entree. Have a healthy salad and a portion of fresh fruit or canned fruit in natural juice.

- ☐ **ENGLISH MUFFIN:** 1 English muffin spread with small amount of fruit spread and skim cottage cheese.

- ☐ **ROLL:** 1 small pumpernickel roll with 1 slice American cheese, reduced fat, and 11/2 cups diced watermelon, in zipper lock bag.

- ☐ **PANCAKES:** Cooked and refrigerated, or freeze; eat at room temperature or heat in a microwave, 3 to 4 pancakes with small amount of fruit spread, 1 hard cooked egg.

- ☐ **BAGEL SANDWICH:** 1 small bagel sandwich, 1 slice cheese reduced fat, 1 fresh apple

- ☐ **BRAN FLAKES:** 1 cup bran flakes (carry in small container with lid), 1 small banana, ½ to ¾ cups low-fat milk

- ☐ **BRAN MUFFIN:** With 1 slice cheese, reduced fat, ½ cup diced fresh pineapple, in zipper lock bag

SNACKING IS A NECESSARY PART OF HEALTHY EATING, WEIGHT LOSS AND MAINTENANCE

SNACKING TO RAISE METABOLISM

Healthy snacking – use foods to lose fat – eat to lose faster. Snacking is not a new concept. Most of us have been doing it but healthy snacking is a key to weight loss and maintenance. For many of us we are always too busy to sit down and eat main meals; snacking on small meals will prevent us from getting too hungry. Snacking may also be necessary to get those nutrients that are missed from skipping meals. Low fat to non-fat snacks are the key. Choose snacks that provide protein, complex carbohydrates, vitamins, and minerals. Snacks must be planned; calories and fat must be kept in mind. Many of the snacks we eat contain 10 or more grams of fat. Look for lower-fat snacks that contain 3 grams or less of fat per serving. Changing snacking habits will take some research on your behalf. You must be aware of the nutrition content of the foods you snack on so it is necessary to read labels for ingredient and nutrient content for fat, sugar, and sodium. It is okay at times to eat your favorite regular snack but it may be better to only eat half. Snacking is recommended to prevent you from getting hungry, which may cause overeating and weight gain.

EATING SMALLER MEALS ARE BETTER

Eating smaller meals throughout the day may be better, instead of the three meals a day pattern. After you eat, your body will release the hormone called insulin. When we consume a large meal that is high in fat and sugar, more insulin is released. The insulin that is released causes the body to save fat and burn carbohydrates. The insulin level is lower and more stable with smaller and more frequent meals. There will be less insulin in the blood, less fat will be stored, and the body will burn fat faster. If necessary, bring your healthy snacks to work so you will not be tempted by the fattening foods.

LOW CALORIE SNACKING

I do not believe in counting calories, but this will give you a guide for healthy snacking. Trace calories per serving. The following snacks are good plain or with a fat-free dressing or homemade dip:

- Celery sticks

- Cucumbers

- Lettuce

- Green peppers

- Cauliflower

- Broccoli

- Greens

- Mushrooms

- Spinach

25-30 calories per serving:

- 1 small tangerine

- ½ cup watermelon, cubed

- ½ cup cantaloupe, cubed

- 1 small tomato

- 1 cup popcorn, no added fat

- ½ cup pretzel sticks

35-40 calories per serving:

- ☐ 1 medium peach

- ☐ 1 medium nectarine

- ☐ ½ grapefruit

- ☐ ½ cup skim milk

- ☐ ¼ cup plain yogurt

- ☐ 3 saltine crackers

- ☐ ½ small banana

50-70 calories per serving:

- ☐ 1 small apple

- ☐ 1 small orange

- ☐ 15 grapes

- ☐ 12 cherries

- ☐ 2 tbsp. raisins

- ☐ ¾ ounce tortilla chips

- ☐ 1 cup strawberries

- ☐ ¼ cup cottage cheese

- ☐ 6 oz. ginger ale

- ☐ 2 oz. or 8 large shrimp (boil, steam or broil)

- ☐ ¼ cup plain pudding

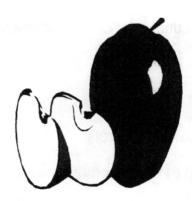

80-100 calories per serving:

- ☐ ¾ cup frozen yogurt

- ☐ 1 cup skim milk plain yogurt

- ☐ ¼ cup sherbet, any flavor

- ☐ 6 each saltine crackers

- ☐ 8 each animal cookies

- ☐ 3 each graham crackers

- ☐ 3 cups popcorn no added fat

- ☐ 2 cups popcorn w/tsp. small amount of butter

- ☐ ½ cup Snack Pack Fat Free Pudding

- ☐ ½ cup regular gelatin

MORE HEALTHY SNACKS. STOP COUNTING CALORIES:

- Reduced fat crackers with fruit spread

- Celery stick stuffed with reduced fat or non-fat cheese spread or reduced fat
  cream cheese

- Skim milk or 1% milk with fresh apple

- Thin apple slices with slice fresh carrots

- Raisins with small amount of peanuts (nuts per serving 10)

- Raisins and a small amount of nuts mixed with plain low fat vanilla yogurt

- Plain tuna fish 1½ ounce mixed with chopped green salad or other vegetables
  make a nice snack

- Half a chicken sandwich (1 oz. white meat, whole wheat toast)

- Mini pizza with reduced fat cheese

- Homemade pizza made with mini bagel or English muffin topped with small
  amount of reduced fat shredded cheese, tomato and diced vegetables may be added

- Pita bread pockets stuffed with chopped or diced tomatoes, diced cucumber, shredded lettuce and shredded low fat or non-fat cheese; may reduce cheese and add 1 ounce shredded white turkey meat, with reduced fat or non-fat dressing.
- Pita bread stuffed with one diced hard boiled egg, shredded or diced lettuce, tomato, cucumber with reduced fat or no fat dressing.

MORE SNACKS:

Eating snacks helps you keep from getting too hungry. A healthy snack is one that is low in fat or about 2 to 3 grams per serving and contains about 15 grams of carbohydrates.

- ☐ Fresh fruit
- ☐ 3 pieces of dried fruit
- ☐ 2 cups raisins
- ☐ 2 fig bars
- ☐ 2 oatmeal-raisin cookies
- ☐ 2 rice cakes
- ☐ 2 bread sticks
- ☐ 1 slice of bread with reduced fat peanut butter
- ☐ ½ cup of cereal with skim milk or 1% milk
- ☐ 1 English muffin with fruit spread
- ☐ 1 cup of low fat or non-fat yogurt
- ☐ 1 cup of reduced fat soup
- ☐ ½ cup fruit juice

- ☐ ½ bagel with reduced fat cottage cheese vegetable spread (homemade)

- ☐ ½ bagel with fruit spread and peanut butter

- ☐ 6 crackers with low fat cheese and grapes

- ☐ 4 ginger snap cookies with cup of tea

- ☐ 1 ounce low fat Tostitos

- ☐ 3 spiced wafer cookies

- ☐ 10 pretzels

- ☐ ½ pita bread with chopped lettuce and tomato with fat-free dressing

SNACKING AND SLEEPING:

Healthy snacking may help you to sleep better. Nighttime snacks will also prevent the next day binges and will provide you with more energy. Night snacking will also keep the metabolism system working, which will cause fat and calorie burning.

PORTION SIZE:

Eating low fat foods does not give you a green light to eat more. If an item is 3 to 5 ounces a portion by eating 2 or more portions can cause problems with total fat or total calories in the long run.

Eating continually is not the problem and to push yourself away from the table is not the answer either. To lose weight and to keep it off, knowing what to eat most of the time, is a must.

You must eat to lose weight when you eat more often, your metabolism will increase. Your metabolism must also rise for digestion. The higher the metabolism rate, the faster calories will be burned.

FIBER

FIBER IS A MISSING LINK FOR HEALTHY EATING AND WEIGHT LOSS

You have heard of fiber or known as roughage. Fiber is a missing link for weight loss and maintenance. Do not even think of starting a healthy eating program without increasing your fiber intake. If you don't, you will be setting yourself up for failure. High fiber foods are filling and it will take longer for you to become hungry again. By eating a variety of foods higher in fiber will make you fuller and you will stay satisfied longer. You will find that by eating foods higher in fiber that smaller portions will fill you up. Your calorie intake will be reduced and you will lose weight and maintain the new weight loss better. The emphasis is to eat more dietary fiber, lower in saturated fat and to reduce your refined sugar intake. The key is to eat more complex carbohydrates, all of which contain both soluble and insoluble fiber to some degree. It is necessary to have both soluble and insoluble fiber for good health. The average American eats only 10-15 grams of fiber daily. It is not necessary to start counting fiber grams, just eat more food from the list provided.

In America our food is highly processed. Much of the dietary fiber that is present in grains and products has been removed. Not only has dietary fiber been removed but much of the vitamin and mineral content has also been lost.

Manufacturers today are producing more grain products that have not gone through the milling process (the removing of roughage or dietary fiber), such as oats, wheat and bran, barley, brown rice, millet and corn. So eat and enjoy more unrefined high-fiber foods. It will take less to fill you up and it will slow down the on set of hunger.

TOO MUCH FIBER TO FAST MAY CAUSE PROBLEMS

Eating too much fiber at the start and if you are not used to high fiber intake can overwhelm the bacteria in the large intestine and may cause excess gas which can also be painful and can also cause constipation or diarrhea.

Start off by eating smaller amounts of fiber at a time, then increase to larger intakes. Do this gradually over several weeks. This will give your stomach a chance to get accustomed to the higher level.

Eat slowly and chew fiber foods well. This will help avoid digestive problems. If over the age of 65 or if you have had gastrointestinal surgery, check with your physician before increasing your intake.

SHOPPING – READ THE PACKAGE FOR FIBER CONTENT

Buy foods high in fiber. Check the labels.

- 2.5 to 4.9 grams of fiber per serving is a good source
- 5 grams of fiber or more per serving (foods high in fiber)

DIETARY FIBER

What is dietary fiber? It is the material from plant cells that we cannot digest or can only partially digest. Fiber also is referred to as roughage, which helps, promotes a healthy digestive tract and prevents constipation. Fiber comes in two forms, soluble and insoluble.

SOLUBLE FIBER – dissolves to a gummy texture during digestion, which slows the absorption.

GOOD SOURCE OF SOLUBLE FIBER

- Dried beans, peas and lentils

- Oatmeal

- Rice bran

- Barley

- Cauliflower, corn

- Apples, pears, strawberries

BENEFIT OF SOLUBLE FIBER:

- Decreases blood cholesterol

- Helps prevent heart disease

- Helps regulate blood sugar

INSOLUBLE FIBER – passes through the digestive system without dissolving.

Good source of insoluble fiber:

- Bran cereals

- Whole wheat bread

- Dried beans

- Popcorn

- Fruit with skin

- Corn

- Broccoli

- Potatoes with skin

BENEFITS OF INSOLUBLE FIBER

- Provide bulk

- Helps the digestive system work properly

- Helps prevent constipation

- Helps prevent hemorrhoids and other intestinal problems

- May lower the risk of some types of cancer

BREAKFAST, SNACKS AND FIBER

Higher fiber breakfast and snacks also help to curb the appetite and help prevent overeating between meals because the onset of hunger will decrease. Also, most high fiber foods are high in vitamin and mineral and lower in fat.

WATER AND FIBER

Drink more water or other low calorie fluids. This will increase the efficiency of the increased fiber intake and will help to prevent the possibility of intestinal obstructions. By drinking more water you will help keep the added fiber moving through your system.

HOW TO ADD MORE FIBER

These foods are more filling and not high in calorie. It is how you prepare these foods. Avoid high fat toppings.

- whole grain bread in place of white

- popcorn as a snack, low fat

- brown rice in place of white

- whole wheat toast

- whole fruits and fruits with skin

- potato with skin

- dried fruits

- vegetables with skin

- nuts and seeds

- legumes (beans and peas) 3 times a week (in casseroles, salads, soups)

- vegetables and vegetables with skin

- mixed vegetable salads

- high fiber breakfast cereals with or without fruit

- whole wheat flour for baking

- all bran (use to thicken dishes, or as a topping on baked vegetables and pasta dishes)

- add all bran to yogurt and as a topping on fruit dishes

- add all bran to whole wheat flour to make baked bread, cake and pie crust (add up to ½ cup of all bran to 4 cups of whole wheat flour)

- whole wheat flour, whole wheat semolina, bran to thicken gravy and sauce

- whole wheat pancakes in place of white

- puree fruit drink with skin

- dried fruits baked in cake and desserts

- stewed fruits with skin

- add legumes, grains, vegetables, and fruits to casseroles and other baked goods

- fruits baked in homemade bread

- fruits, sorbets or shakes (puree fruit with skin)

- angel food cake topped with diced mixed fresh fruits or fruit pureed with skin

WAYS TO CHANGE YOUR RECIPES INTO HIGHER FIBER

1.   Add cooked beans and peas to soups, stews, casseroles and salads.

2.   Add nuts and seeds to salads as topping for desserts, add to baked bread and rice pudding. Mix into puddings, yogurts and various desserts. Try adding nuts and seeds to other dishes, like rice, pasta and vegetables.

3.   Cut back on meat at least one or two times a week. Serve a meal made with dried beans or peas. There are many cookbooks for vegetarian meals.

4.   Leave the skin on potatoes and other vegetables if possible.

5.   Add fresh or dried fruits to desserts, casseroles or salads. Leave skin on when adding to recipe if possible. (stewed apples or pears with skin)

6.   Make home baked bread high in fiber (whole grain flour) wheat pancakes

7.   In recipes in place of white rice use brown rice or white pasta use whole wheat pasta

EXAMPLE OF RECIPE SUBSTITUTION TO INCREASE FIBER

1 cup all-purpose flour, substitute the following:

-   1 cup finely milled whole wheat flour

-   ¾ cup white flour and ¼ cup bran

-   7/8 cup coarsely milled whole wheat flour

FOOD WITH HIGH FIBER CONTENT

1.   Bread and Crackers

     rye bread
     whole wheat   *100% whole wheat flour
     pumpernickel bread/rolls
     muffins: bran, oat, corn, and graham crackers
     triscuits
     rye krisp

whole wheat matzo
whole wheat pita
whole wheat english muffin
whole wheat bagel
corn tortillas

2.   Cereals

all bran-extra fiber
fiber-one
all-bran, fruits and almonds
100% bran
bran buds
bran chex
corn bran
cracklin' oat bran
bran flakes
grapenuts
air-popped popcorn
wheat germ
shredded wheat
total
wheaties
wheat chex
muffets, wheat
puffed wheat
corn flakes
raisin bran
wheatena
whole wheat farina
oatmeal
rolled oats
scotch oats
coarsely ground cornmeal
barley, whole grain
bulgur
buckwheat
cuscous
cornmeal, stone ground
guinoa
whole grain, flour wheat
rye, buckwheat
whole wheat pasta

*all bran 40% bran
*unprocessed or miller's bran
*granola type cereals

oats, and brains. Choose less often products made with refined flours – white breads,

rolls, pastries, and cakes.

4.   Cooked Legumes

      kidney beans
      vegetarian beans, baked
      lentils
      pinto beans
      black northern beans
      navy beans
      green peas
      yellow split pea
      black eye

5.   Fruits

      apple
      apricots
      banana
      cherries
      peaches
      prunes, plum
      strawberries
      nectarine
      blackberries
      blueberries
      pomegranate
      raspberries
      mulberries
      currants
      apple with skin
      apricots
      cherries
      grapes
      grapefruit
      kumquats
      melon
      nectarines
      oranges
      peaches
      pears
      plums
      tangerines
      tangelos

raisins
dates
pineapple raisins

6.   Vegetables

     wax beans
     green beans
     broccoli
     brussel sprouts
     cabbage
     carrots
     cauliflower
     corn
     lettuce
     onions
     parsnips
     green peas
     potato with skin
     spinach
     tomatoes
     turnips

*Choose from among all the fruits and vegetables, both fresh and frozen.

Miscellaneous:

peanuts, roasted with skin
peanut butter
marmalade
pickles

LEGUMES

BEANS PROVIDE AN EXCELLENT SOURCE OF COMPLEX CARBOHYDRATES AND ARE LOW IN FAT, LOW CALORIES, FULL OF PROTEIN, AND A GOOD SOURCE OF FIBER

Beans are a dietary staple for millions of people throughout the world.

Beans provide an excellent source of complex carbohydrates. You will need about 4 to 5 slices of wheat bread to equal ½ cup of soybeans or navy beans.

Although beans are a good source of protein, they are missing one or two essential amino acids (amino acids are the building blocks of protein).

Beans are not complete in essential amino acids but they are an excellent source of protein when combined with grains, nuts or seeds. Beans can also be combined with a small amount of meat, fish, or reduced fat cheese and other dairy products. When beans are eaten in combination with the above products, the added items will provide complete protein or essential amino acids.

Beans are a good source of fiber. Cooked beans provide between 10-15 grams of fiber per cup. Beans contain both soluble and insoluble fiber, which will help curb hunger. We want to eat more foods low in calorie, low in fat, and low in cholesterol. Add more beans to your meal plan and you will not only lose weight but also maintain your ideal body weight.

Beans are a good source of iron, calcium, vitamins, zinc, magnesium, potassium, and phosphorus. When eating fruits and vegetables that are high in vitamin C along with beans, iron absorption is increased.

TO HELP PREVENT GAS

Beans that are less likely to cause gas are black-eyed peas, chick peas, lentil beans, lima beans, white beans, and soybean products like tofu and tempeh. Follow these directions to reduce gas for all types of beans:

1. Discard water that is used to soak beans.

2. Take a few drops of Beano before eating beans or other gassy foods. (Note: Beano comes in both liquid and tablets and may be of help in preventing gas).

3. Eat beans in smaller amounts, and add more to your meal plan as you go along.

4.   Do not eat beans with other foods that may cause you gas.

NOTE: The following complex carbohydrate foods may cause gas but they are also good fat burning foods, so with Beano, they may not produce as much gas: beans, cabbage, cauliflower, broccoli, whole grains and pasta, onions, and some soy foods.

SOYBEANS

RESEARCH SHOWS THAT FLAVONES (PLANT HORMONES CALLED PHYTOESTROGENS) IN SOYBEANS MAY HELP REDUCE RISK OF:

1.   Osteoporosis (bone loss)

2.   Breast cancer

3.   Prostate cancer

4.   Reduce total blood cholesterol (if greater than 260 mg./dl)

5.   Reduce LDL-cholesterol

6.   Reduce menopausal symptoms

SUGAR AND WEIGHT LOSS AND MAINTENANCE – SIMPLE CARBOHYDRATE

If you want to control your weight, it is necessary to control your sugar intake. Sugar reducing tips will reduce unnecessary calories. By reducing your sugar intake, you will be decreasing the total caloric intake. It is not necessary to cut out sugar all together, only cut back. Many of us add additional sugar to the food and we eat them in the form of sugar itself, or as jelly, syrup, honey, etc.

Serve naturally-sweet desserts such as fresh fruits. Used canned fruit packed in natural juice or light syrup. Serve jello with lower calorie whip topping. Serve instant pudding made with skim milk or 1% milk and less sugar. You may serve jello or pudding with unsweetened canned or fresh fruit. Serve plain non-fat yogurt with fresh or canned unsweetened fruit, this makes a nice healthy dessert.

Instead of serving syrup over pancakes, waffles, or French toast, top with applesauce, fresh fruit, fruit spread, stewed, chilled, cooked fruit or syrup with half the sugar.

Bananas or raisins may be used in baking as a sweetener in place of sugar. Orange slices or raisins may be used as a sweetener in place of sugar. Try adding orange slices and raisins to yams and sweet potatoes instead of sugar or regular syrup. Try adding raisins to plain cold cereal and hold or cut back on the sugar.

Serve fruit spread on muffins, bagels, toast, English muffins, etc., instead of jelly or jam. This will reduce calories. When sugar is used in recipes, cut the sugar by 1/3. This will save on calories.

SUGAR , CONCENTRATED SWEET AND WEIGHT GAIN

Sugar is known to be a main cause of obesity. The average American consumes about 30 to 40 teaspoons of sugar a day. There has been an increase in obesity in this country because of the sugar intake from the foods and drinks that are being chosen by people each day. Many people are overweight not because they eat too much, but because they may eat too much of the wrong foods like (cake, cookies, soft drinks, or high fat foods)

Sugar and concentrated sweets should be avoided during weight loss. Try to avoid too much sweets as much as possible, eat them in moderation. Also many sugary foods are high in fat and low in vitamins and minerals. Reduce the intake of concentrated sweets or refined carbohydrates to control your caloric intake. You must get more of your calories from more complex carbohydrates that have nutritional value (vitamins, minerals, and fiber). Increase your intake of whole grain bread and cereals, fresh fruits and vegetables.

SUGAR AND EXERCISE

Never consume sugar after you exercise because you are working out to burn fat. If you eat or drink sugar right after your workout, the sugar will be burned first.

FOODS HIGH IN SUGAR MUST BE USED IN MODERATION

Sugar is a carbohydrate. It is one of the two types of carbohydrates. Sugar is a simple carbohydrate. It is half as many calories as fat, but is known to cause weight gain and it also provides what is known as empty calories. It has no vitamins, minerals, or other nutrients. You want as many nutrients as possible from the foods you eat especially when the amount of calories is reduced for weight loss and maintenance.

READ YOUR FOOD LABELS

Sugar is added to almost all processed foods in some amount if you read your food labels in the packages. If sugar such as sucrose, glucose, dextrose, maltose, lactose, fructose, or syrup appear at or near the top of the list, you may not want to stock too many of these foods in your pantry. Remember when you want to eat or cook, you will properly use the foods or ingredients already stores in your pantry or refrigerator first. Try to stock more healthy foods.

SECTION – B

Section-B formally supports the knowledge you gain from Section-A. It plays an important role in providing you with the necessary information to support what you have put into motion by assisting you in staying focus on your primary goals of eating healthier for life and managing your weight. Some changes are necessary and you are provided with some easy life style techniques and activities. It is mainly up to you, by now you should know that there is no quick fix.

I am going out of my mind looking for a quick fix. There must be missing links.

Very Low Calorie Diet

Soup Diet

Diet Pills

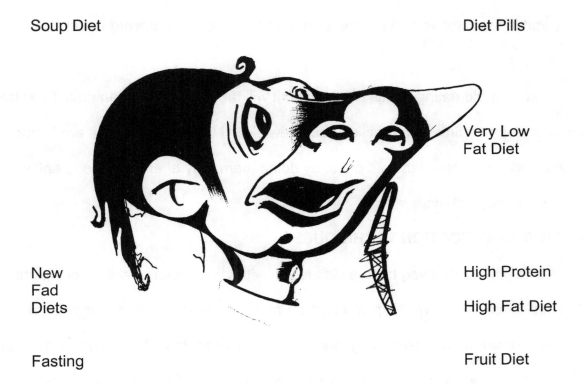

Very Low
Fat Diet

New
Fad
Diets

High Protein

High Fat Diet

Fasting

Fruit Diet

Vegetable Diet

Confused about what diets work? Stay away from diets that promise quick weight loss. Most do no work and some can be extremely dangerous.

There is no quick fix.

BEHAVIOR MODIFICATION:

Behavior modification is a big term that means, simply, changing the things that you do. Eating is a behavior. You learned how, when, and what to eat as you were growing up. Your parents, your friends, and your spouse all helped teach you. If you are overweight, the chances are that at least some of these eating behaviors, or habits, are not working well for you. It is time for a change – a change toward better, healthier ways to eat.

Changing old eating habits is easy and it will take work. You can do it if you take things one step at a time and practice each new skill. New healthy habits are learned the same way you learned the old ones: by doing them, day after day. Good eating habits include good choices.

BEHAVIOR MODIFICATION TECHNIQUES:

1. It is important that you have a discussion with your doctor, dietitian, or weight loss coach. They will help you plan a program specially tailored for you, taking into consideration many things that are particular to you. It is important that you eat three well-balanced meals per day plus low calorie snacks in order to stay mentally and physically healthy and at your best.

2. In order for any weight reduction efforts to work for you, first examine why you eat. It is possible that if you eat for the wrong reasons, you may be able to modify the behavior. Identify the reasons: Boredom, anxiety, tension, depression, worry, frustration, avoiding disturbing relationships or activities, or to show love or affection for another person. It is suggested that if you eat for these reasons that you find some activity to do, other than eating. It is also important

that you identify the time of the day that is the greatest temptation for you: mid-morning, afternoon, or evening. During the time of day you are more tempted to eat, stay busy.

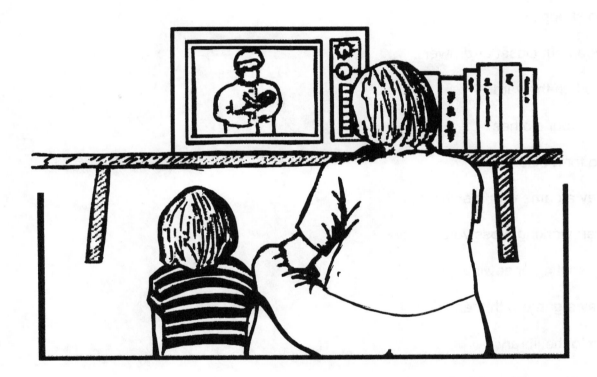

ACTIVITIES YOU CAN DO IN PLACE OF EATING WHEN BOREDOM, ANXIETY, TENSION, DEPRESSION, WORRYING, AND FRUSTRATION SET IN:

Examples are given below for activities that can be substituted for eating. Review this list regularly in order to keep these activities in mind for use, as needed.

- ☐ Walk the dog
- ☐ Clean the house
- ☐ Go shopping
- ☐ Clean out closet or drawer
- ☐ Work in the yard
- ☐ Iron your clothes
- ☐ Go for a bike ride
- ☐ Play a game with the children
- ☐ Start working crossword puzzles
- ☐ Do knitting or sewing
- ☐ Play a game with friends
- ☐ Go to the library
- ☐ Rearrange the furniture
- ☐ Do your laundry
- ☐ Fix something that is broken in the house
- ☐ Go somewhere you have never been
- ☐ Give your friend a call
- ☐ Take a bath
- ☐ Go to a movie

- ☐   Play a game of cards

- ☐   Start a hobby

- ☐   Listen to the radio

- ☐   Write a letter

- ☐   Go for a swim

- ☐   Trim the yard

- ☐   Water the plant

- ☐   Clean the car

- ☐   Check garage sales

BEHAVIOR MODIFICATION TECHNIQUES – HELP PREVENT OVEREATING

- Store food out of sight.

- Keep lower fat, lower calorie foods on hand.

- Use smaller plates to serve food.

- Concentrate on eating slower, chew your food longer before swallowing. This will give you a feeling of fullness.

- Preplan meals for two or three days ahead.

- Use smaller or more shallows soup or cereal bowls.

- Pace yourself to 20 minutes to half an hour to eat. Really taste the food and get the pleasure out of the food.

- Keep serving dishes off the table, you may be tempted to eat more.

- Do not store high fat foods or your favorite high fat foods in the house or in the office.

- Do not skip breakfast.

- Get regular sleep, tiredness often leads to overeating to gain energy.

- Eat small portions of snacks more often to prevent hunger.

- Eat lower fat snacks between meals.

- Do not use food as a reward.

- Do not eat more than one or two high fat higher calorie meals in a week.

- Choose lower calorie snacks that are more filling. An apple is more filling than apple juice.

BEHAVIOR MODIFICATION TO BURN FAT AND CALORIES

- Walk more outside or inside .

- Do more physical activity. Example – clean the house, work in the garden, etc.

- Do more activities like swimming, bowling, hiking, biking, etc.

- Join the gym or health club.

- Walk up the stairs whenever possible.

- Park the car a few blocks away and walk to work.

- Get off the bus a few stops away and walk back.

- Hire a personal trainer for support.

- Dance around the house.

BEHAVIOR MODIFICATION TECHNIQUES–DINING OUT ON SPECIAL OCCASIONS

- Eat fewer calories early in the week, the total calorie for the week is more important than the total calorie for the day.

- You can ask the restaurants if they will serve you a lower fat, low sugar menu or, you can eat your favorite foods when dining out but just eat less and take the remainder home for the portions are usually larger

- Eat slowly and enjoy the food.

- Eat a light snack before going to a special party or when dining out.

- Eat a snack about ½ hour before having that holiday meal.

- If you over eat on some occasions like on Thanksgiving, etc., it's okay just go back to healthier eating the next day

- When you find yourself going out a lot during the holidays, make sure to carry with you some low fat snacks so you can snack before going to big events.

- Avoid the cocktail hour or just eat less and do not stand near the food.

- Avoid high calorie beverages.

- When dining out, ask the waiter to serve all sauces, gravy, butter, etc. on the side.

- Do cut back on high calorie desserts or have half the amount on the holiday itself, just enjoy yourself.

- Try to eat more fresh fruits during the holidays.

- Do not go to the party early especially when buffet is being served.

BEHAVIOR MODIFICATION – AWARENESS – CAUSES OF OBESITY

In order for any weight reduction to work, you need to know what is causing your weight problem. List the 5 main causes of weight gain.

1._____

2._____

3._____

4._____

5._____

ANSWER TO (5) FIVE MAIN CAUSES OF OBESITY:

1.   Overeating

2.   Lack of Activity

3.   Abnormalities of Glandular Functioning

4.   Emotional Problems

5.   Genetics

CAUSES OF OBESITY:

Obesity is caused by an intake of calories beyond the body's need for energy. The two main causes of obesity are overeating and the lack of activity.

1.   **Overeating:** is one of the main causes of obesity. Some people continue to gain weight throughout life because they fail to adjust their eating habits to their reduced calorie requirements as they get older. These unchanged food habits can cause you to take in more food than is needed. A small amount of food eaten in excess each day will in time cause unwanted weight gain.

2.   **Lack of Activity:** lack of exercise has been said to be one of the most important causes of obesity. As you become older, your physical activity and metabolism usually decrease. If your food habits do not change, your weight will most likely increase. It is necessary to eat less food or to increase your activity, or both, in order to keep your weight down.

OTHER CAUSES OF OBESITY:

1.   **Abnormalities of glandular functioning:** Glandular conditions are rarely the

cause of obesity. Glandular and other physiological problems are only responsible for 1% to 2% of all cases of obesity or overweight.

2. **Emotional problems:** can contribute to overweight. Some people will overeat due to frustration, to relive tension, depression, or they are just plain bored. At times, the obese state may be the protective resolution of deeper emotional problems.

3. **Fat and genetics:** Obese children are more likely than non-obese children to be obese adults. Surveys show that where one parent of a child is obese, about 40% of the offspring are obese. When both parents are obese, 80% of the offspring are obese. If your parents are overweight or obese, this may increase your chances of being obese too. Your genes may make it easier for you to be overweight by 25% to 30%.

REGAINING WEIGHT:

95% of people who lose weight will regain the weight back within 5 years. When the weight is regained, it will add more fat cells to your body and it will become harder for you to lose the weight the second, third, etc., time around.

BEHAVIOR MODIFICATION – EATING FOR THE WRONG REASONS:

It is possible that you eat for the wrong reasons. You may be able to modify your behavior. Write down as many reasons you feel you are eating for the wrong reasons.

_____

_____

_____

_____

BEHAVIOR MODIFICATION – ACTIVITIES

If you eat for the wrong reasons, you need to find some other activities to do other than eating. List as many activities you can do in place of eating.

_____

_____

_____

_____

_____

_____

_____

I KNOW I LOOK GOOD

Improper dieting can cause the breakdown of lean muscle mass. A person can lose weight and be thin and still have a high body fat percentage.

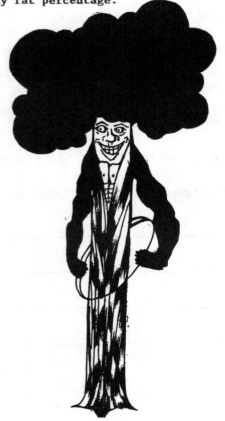

FAT, PROTEIN, CARBOHYDRATE

Eat smart. If any nutrients are missing the body may not grow or develop properly.

A BALANCE OF ALL NUTRIENTS IS NECESSARY

Eating a variety of foods is important. The so called fad diets that omit one food group which provide essential nutrients that is needed for the body to function can cause other health problems. With the omission of one nutrient, the other nutrient or nutrients may need to be increased to provide needed calories. You

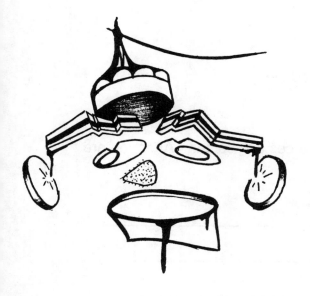

must avoid any diet that is high only in one nutrient (high protein, high fat, or high carbohydrate. When a diet is extremely high in one nutrient and extremely low in another, you may be putting your health into jeopardy. Example: The high protein diet restricts the nutrient carbohydrate extremely which will cause the consumption of excessive amount of protein and fat which can also cause harm on vital organs.

YOU CANNOT OMIT ANY NUTRIENTS FOR HEALTHY EATING OR WEIGHT LOSS

For the body to function properly, you need to eat all the nutrients in a correct portion. Eat a well-balanced meal plan which consist of a variety of foods from the food groups in moderation.

FAT – A meal plan that is too low in fat will not work for weight loss and maintenance. More fat is allowed. The recommendation of total fat % in each meal has increased from 25% and 30% fat to 35% fat. The increased recommended fat must come from unsaturated fat. I have always and still recommend no less than 30% to 35% fat. The higher recommended fat % range is to help people stick with a healthier eating pattern for life. Fat increase palatability of food and provide satiety and delay onset of hunger making it easier for many people to stay with healthier eating habits.

FAT – NUTRIENT – FUNCTIONS:

1.   Provide energy

2.   Carries fat-soluble vitamins – A, D, E, K

3.   Provides essential fatty acids the body cannot produce

4.   Helps form membranes

Test your knowledge of fats. List as many fat sources as you can. After you are done, turn the page to note it.

_____

_____

_____

_____

_____

_____

_____

_____

_____

_____

_____

_____

_____

_____

FAT SOURCES:

1. Oil

2. Butter

3. Margarine

4. Cooking fats

5. Mayonnaise

6. Most cheeses

7. Whole milk

8. Egg yolk

9. Peanut butter

10. Nuts

11. Chocolate

12. Coconut

13. Fatty meats

14. Fried foods

15. There are also hidden fats in foods like cream sauces, salad dressings, gravy, quick bread, muffins, and snack foods.

FATS PLACE IN A HEALTHIER MEAL PLAN

CUTTING BACK ON FAT (BUT SOME FAT IS NECESSARY)

Cutting back on total fat can help you prevent or treat obesity and other health problems. Restricting one particular type of fat (saturated fat) is the key.

Fat contains more than twice as many calories as either carbohydrates or protein. Calories we eat from fat are easily converted to body fat than other sources of calories (protein and carbohydrates).

Fat requires little energy to turn it to body fat (about 3 percent, as opposed to 25 percent for carbohydrates). The consumption of all fats must be controlled to prevent weight gain and other diseases. If you cut calories, you should also cut fat.

WE DO NEED SOME FAT

Some fat is necessary. Our body needs fat to function properly. Fat is necessary to provide a good source of energy. It aids in absorption of fat-soluble vitamins (A, D, E, and K). Some fat sources provide Linoleic Acid, a fatty acid, which is considered essential for good health.

LOWER FAT

Food technology has provided us with many versions of so many foods like ice cream, cheeses, and lower fat meats. Some of these new low fat products taste as good as the original high fat ones. There are thousands of these new foods in the supermarket, health food stores, and served in restaurants. It is up to you to single out the lower fat foods that you enjoy. You must learn to combine lower fat versions and essential fats in moderation; too low fat intake also may cause unwanted health problems too.

THERE ARE TWO MAIN TYPES OF FATS:

1.   Saturated Fat – Saturated fats come from animal sources such as red meat, poultry, fish, and eggs, and dairy products such as butter and cheese. Some saturated fats are from tropical vegetables such as coconut, palm kernel, and palm oils.

Saturated fats are usually solid at room temperature. The body needs some saturated fat but too much saturated fat may raise the level of bad cholesterol (LDL) and lower the level of good cholesterol (HDL). High levels of cholesterol can cause fatty build-up in the walls of the blood vessels. The fatty accumulation can also cause heart disease and strokes. Too much saturated fat is said to cause some forms of cancer.

2.   Unsaturated Fat – Unsaturated fat is known to lower the risk of heart disease, stroke, and some forms of cancer. Unsaturated fats are usually liquid at room temperature and are mainly found in vegetables and plant foods with some vegetable oil. Unsaturated fats are divided into two groups – monounsaturated and polyunsaturated fats. These two groups are good for you but due to the high calories, intake should be in moderation. NOTE: Polyunsaturated fat also contains two essential fatty acids (EFA) that are necessary for the body to function properly: Alpha-Linoleic (LNA) and Linoleic Acid (LA). These fatty acids are the precursors of hormone-like compounds that help regulate the blood pressure, heart rate, blood clotting, central nervous system, immune response, and assists in the body recovery time from physical fatigue. Our bodies do not manufacture essential fatty acids (EFAs). We get them from foods we eat.

- Alpha-Linoleic Acid – which is a form of "Alpha-Omega-3 Fatty Acid" is needed to help decrease the risk of heart disease. It lowers "Bad" cholesterol and will decrease the liver's production of triglycerides. Alpha-Linoleic acid also helps fight osteoporosis by slowing the body's excretion of calcium.

- [] Linoleic Acid – is necessary for healthy hair and skin, and helps to prevent degeneration of the kidneys and liver, and helps fight osteoporosis (the body will be better able to absorb calcium).

- [] Note: Homemade salad dressing by using a combination of oil with the EFAs (Sunflower oil, olive oil, mustard, and walnuts oil, vinegar, or lemon juice).

- [] Other food sources: Side dishes - make a bean or lentil pilaf in place of rice as a side dish and serve with fish. Stir-fry Tofu with vegetables and 1 tablespoon of dark sesame oil.

VEGETABLES OILS HIGH IN EFAs:

Sunflower Oil Safflower Oil Peanut Oil Sesame Oil	These oils are good for high heat cooking (frying)
Canola Oil Corn Oil Sunflower Oil	Medium high heat cooking (baking, sautéing)
Olive Oil Peanut Oil Walnut Oil Soy Oil	Medium heat cooking (light sautéing, sauces)
Flaxseed Oil Canola Oil Olive Oil	Low to no heating (soup, salads)

NATIONAL RESEARCH COUNCIL DAILY RECOMMENDATIONS OF ESSENTIAL FATTY ACIDS (EFAs):

1. Alpha-Linoleic Acid (LNA): Flaxseed, Linseed, or Walnut Oil – 1 to 2 tablespoons daily of oil (high in LNA).

2. Linoleic Acid (LA): Safflower, Sunflower, Corn, Sesame, or Peanut Oil – 1 to 2 teaspoons daily of oil (high in LA).

3.   NOTE – Walnuts have both the essential fatty acids (EFAs) and can be used as a topping for low-fat salads. Dried butternuts and soybeans are good sources of Alpha-Linoleic Acids (LNA). Serve dried butternuts on salad. Add soybeans to stir fry and other main dishes, hot or cold.

HYDROGENATED FAT:

Monounsaturated Fat is found in olive, canola, and peanut oil, and most nuts. Polyunsaturated Fat is found in corn, sunflower, and soybean oil, mayonnaise, and soft margarine. Hydrogenated Fat is a process that turns polyunsaturated oils like corn oil, that are generally liquid at room temperature, into harder, more saturated fats like margarine. Hydrogenation does not make fat completely saturated.

WEIGHT CONTROL AND CHOLESTROL

Cholesterol is not the same as fat. Cholesterol is a waxy substance. To lose or maintain your weight, you may want to eat fewer foods that have a lot of saturated fat and bad cholesterol. On occasions when you eat foods that are high in fat, select foods that have more unsaturated fat. Saturated fats raise your cholesterol level more than anything you eat. Unsaturated fats lower your cholesterol level.

We have been taught that to lower cholesterol levels, simply avoid foods high in cholesterol. We know now that the amount and type of fat we eat will influence our blood cholesterol levels more than the amount of dietary cholesterol eaten. Try to limit your calories from fat. Too much cholesterol is a second cousin to fat. Try to consume 300 mg or less of cholesterol daily. What are the dietary sources of cholesterol? Dietary cholesterol is found only in foods of animal origin.

Eat less total fat, saturated fat (meat, dairy products, and bakery goods raise blood cholesterol more than other fat intake). You will also lower saturated fat and Trans-fatty acids. The more saturated fat you eat, the more cholesterol your body makes. So if you eat lower fat or the right kind of fats in moderation you will be controlling your cholesterol level and also your weight and you will be avoiding other health problems too.

TRANS FATTY ACIDS:

Trans fatty acids are considered harmful, since they may also raise LDL – cholesterol (low-density lipoprotein or "bad" cholesterol, which deposit cholesterol into arteries) and reduce HDL – high-density lipoprotein or "good" cholesterol, which carries cholesterol away from the heart. But Trans fatty acids (found in crackers, cookies, margarine, and partially hydrogenated vegetable oils) may not raise blood cholesterol as much as saturated fat does. More research is needed.

1. Use low fat or non-fat, soft butter or margarine with liquid vegetable oil listed as the first ingredient and less than 2 grams of saturated fat per serving.

2. Use butter that has reduced or no saturated fat and cholesterol.

3. Use monounsaturated fats, which reduce LDLs without lowering HDLs good fat (canola oil, olive oil, avocados, peanuts).

4. Polyunsaturated fat may reduce both LDL and HDL cholesterol. Too much of any oil is unhealthy, so it is necessary to reduce the total fat used in the food preparation.

5. Use margarine or substitutes that read trans fatty acids free.

These products contain a smaller amount of trans-fatty acids, so enjoy them in moderation. Too much can cause weight gain.

Product	Serving	Trans-fatty-acid content
mayonnaise	1 tsp	0.01g
vegetable oil	1 tsp	0.02g
pizza	1 slice	0.13g
potato chips	15 chips	0.11g

COCONUT – SATURATED FAT – AVOID

Use only on special occasions. A serving of coconut is 2 tablespoons. Try cutting back, use 1 to 2 teaspoons per serving.

Note: Try to avoid these saturated fatty foods, eating or in cooking.

Butter, bacon, regular sour cream, regular milk, heavy cream, regular whipped cream, regular cheese, salt port, coconut, but on that special holiday occasion, don't worry, just enjoy. One day should not cause a problem.

CHITTERLINGS – SATURATED FAT – AVOID

Eat only on some occasions like the holidays. Before cooking, clean all visual fat and discard it. Cook for about ½ hour before seasoning. Discard water and wash off fat. Season and complete cooking.

Eat less, serve over rice as a topping and do not spoon out too much sauce over the rice.

FISH: EAT MORE FOR BETTER HEALTH - OMEGA – 3 FATTY ACIDS

Fish is low in saturated fat and cholesterol. Fish contains Omega-3 fatty acids was revealed through research to lower blood triglycerides (fat in blood) and raise HDL (good cholesterol) which is said to reduce heart attack in men by reducing blood clotting.

Omega-3 fatty acid may also reduce blood pressure (risk factors for heart disease) and may also fight the spread of some forms of cancer cells. Studies show that there was 38% lower risk of heart disease and a 60% lower risk of heart attacks than men who did not eat fish.

Eat fish 2 to 3 times a week or at least 7 ounces per week. Researchers at one time recommend only fatty fish (e.g. – mackerel, herring, trout, salmon, herring, sardines, albacore tuna), but all kinds of lean fish such as tuna are also equally beneficial. Avoid fatty meats but do not avoid fatty fish. Fish oil supplements containing Omega-3 fatty acids may not lower blood cholesterol in most people and their safety is questionable (eat fish instead).

EATING YOUR FAVORITE FOODS HIGHER IN FAT - MODERATION IS THE KEY:

Never say never to your favorite high fat foods, but just avoid and cut back or have only on special occasions.

Bacon – Saturated Fat – Avoid

Read the label on the package. Select the leanest. If this is a food you like, let it be that occasional higher fat meal. To say people can never eat bacon and eggs or have a bacon, lettuce and tomato sandwich is so unreal. Try to eat the leaner type, cut the portion from 4 or 3 slices to 2 slices. Eat more often. Lean boiled ham or Canadian bacon or turkey bacon is better. Try lean bacon or lean ham with eggs (two egg whites and only one egg yolk). If you grill or bake bacon on a rack, let the grease drip off. The bacon will be crisp and just as lean as lean boiled ham or Canadian bacon.

PROTEIN – to maintain your weight and for the body to function properly we need to eat the correct amount of protein.

PROTEIN – NUTRIENT FUNCTION:

1.   Build body tissues

2.   Maintain and repair body tissue

3.   Assist with body secretions (enzyme fluid/and hormones)

4.   Helps maintain a proper balance of fluid in some parts of the body

5.   Helps the body fight infection

        Test your knowledge of protein. List as many protein source as you can.

_____

_____

_____

_____

_____

_____

_____

_____

_____

_____

_____

_____

_____

PROTEIN SOURCE:

1. Meat

2. Poultry

3. Fish

4. Eggs

5. Cheese

6. Milk

7. Dried beans

8. Soybeans

9. Peas

10. Nuts

11. Cereals

12. Bread

13. Some vegetables

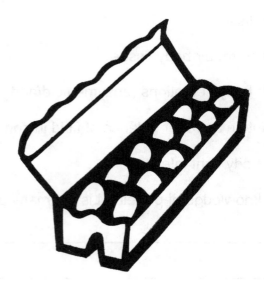

PROTEIN FROM MEAT:

How much protein from meat is enough? The average American eats too much meat. However, meat protein plays a major role in the way the body functions. Protein builds and repairs tissues, enzymes, and antibodies. Meat is an excellent source of vitamin B6 and Zinc. These nutrients can be lacking in an unbalanced vegetarian diet. Meat is also a good source of vitamin B12, which is available only in animal products. Meat is a good source of iron. The body absorbs the iron in meat very well. Too much meat is not good; lean meat also has some saturated fat, which can clog the arteries.

Eating too much protein can also cause a strain on the kidneys. The kidneys excrete protein waste. Too much protein can also decrease the levels of bone-building calcium.

The recommended daily allowance (RDA) from meat is 46 grams for women, and 58 grams for men. You will not be weighing grams of meat, so follow these basic rules: Eat no more than 6 to 7 ounces of lean meat daily, which is not more than two servings of cooked meat. A 3-ounce serving of meat is about the size of a deck of cards.

All your protein sources do not need to come from meat and you do not need to eat only a vegetarian diet to eat lower fat. For weight maintenance, in place of high fat meats, eat lower fat meats more often for healthier eating. You should eat two or three vegetarian meals a week, two to three fish meats a week, but do not stop eating meat.

All our protein sources do not come from meat. Getting your recommended daily allowance (RDA) of protein is easy. Examples:

BREAKFAST	**PROTEIN GRAMS**
1 cup cooked cereal	6
1 cup low fat milk	8
1 small banana	0
Snack:	
1 small apple	0

LUNCH	
Tuna and fresh salad tossed with	
reduced fat dressing (2 ounces	
tuna and 1 cup raw vegetables)	14
1 bagel	6

DINNER	PROTEIN GRAMS
3 ounces lean steak, broiled	21
1 small baked potato	3
1 cup steamed carrots	4
Snack:	
6 crackers	3
4 ounces low-fat milk	<u>4</u>
TOTAL PROTEIN GRAMS:	**69 grams**

COMPLEX CARBOHYDRATES: are necessary for a healthy weight loss and maintenance.

CARBOHYDRATES- NUTRITION – FUNCTION

1.   Principle source of energy

2.   Needed for Elimination

3.   Intestinal system health

4.   Assist the body to use fat efficiently

Test your knowledge of carbohydrate. List as many carbohydrates as you can.

_____

_____

_____

_____

_____

_____

_____

CARBOHYDRATE – SOURCE

1.   Grains

2.   Bread

3.   Cereal

4.   Pasta (macaroni, noodles, spaghetti)

5.   Rice

6.   Corn

7.   Dried beans

8.   Baked goods (cake, cookies, etc.)

9.   Legumes

10.   Potatoes

11.   Nuts and seeds

12.   Bananas and other fruits

13.   Sugar

14.   Syrup

15.   Jams and jellies

16.   Honey

17.   Frosting

18.   Other sweets

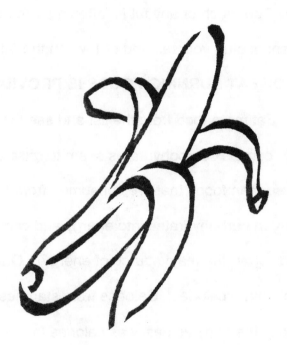

SOME COMPLEX CARBOHYDRATES ARE SAID TO BE

FAT BURNING FOODS – EAT MORE

Researchers have identified some complex carbohydrates as fat burning foods. You should eat more of these foods but avoid adding fatty toppings. Use lower fat or no fat toppings.

Example: Pasta and olive oil. Place olive oil in a spray bottle and spray over the pasta. Too much of any fat is fattening. You can eat more on the list provided but you still cannot stuff yourself and still watch the fatty toppings and fatty ingredients.

LIST OF FAT BURNING FOODS IS PROVIDED

Eat more food from the list and see the difference in your weight. Foods that are high in complex carbohydrates seem to raise the metabolic rates of overweight people more so than foods that are consumed from fats and proteins. It is easier for the body to convert carbohydrates into energy and carbohydrates break down easily into glucose (blood sugar, the main source of energy). Our body prefers to fuel itself with carbohydrate calories. Calories from starches, sugar, and other carbohydrates are not stored in the body as easily as calories from fat.

Research shows that the body converts carbohydrates into energy faster and fat is converted into body fat for future needs.

Dietary fat is similar in chemical composition to the body fat and takes less energy to convert it for storage. Too much fat storage can cause a person to become overweight, which can cause other health problems

COMPLEX CARBOHYDRATES FOODS ARE NOT FATTENING, BUT DRESSING UP

WHEN PREPARING ANY FOODS WITH INGREDIENTS HIGH IN FAT AND SUGER

WILL TAKE ANY FOODS OUT OF A HEALTY RANGE.

LIST OF FAT BURNING FOODS

(HIGH IN COMPLEX CARBOHYDRATES AND LOW IN FAT)

FRUITS

apples	tangerine	pineapples
bananas	cranberries	lemon
grapefruit	cantaloupes	lime
nectarines	honeydew melons	peaches
oranges	dates	prunes
blackberries	figs	raspberries
blueberries	pears	strawberries

VEGETABLES – DURING WEIGHT LOSE EAT MORE OF THESE VEGETABLES

green beans	celery	bell peppers
wax beans	corn	white potatoes
Italian beans	leeks	sweet potatoes (yams)
broccoli	lettuce	red potatoes
cabbage, red, white	mushrooms	spinach
cauliflower	green peas	
tomatoes	zucchini	

ROOTS – VEGETABLES

rutabagas
turnips
parsnips
beets
taro

OTHER HEALTHY VEGETABLES

asparagus	kale
beet greens	kohlrabi
bok choy	mustard green
brussels sprout	pumpkin
carrots	radish green
collard greens	water cress
dandelion green	
garden crest	

FAT BURNING FOODS

white
whole wheat
rye
pumpernickle
French
Italian
bagel
plan bread sticks
plan croutons
English muffin

frankfurter bun
plain burger bun
pita bread
plain matzoh
plain roll
saltine type crackers
oyster crackers
pancakes
waffles

PART OF BREAD GROUP

pasta
white rice
brown rice
all bran
bran buds
bran flakes
shredded wheat
wheat germ
barley
back wheat

bulger wheat
corn bran
corn meal
oat bran
oatmeal
rice bran
wheat bran

LEGUMES

kidney beans
navy beans
white beans
split peas
lima beans
lentils
black-eye peas (cow peas)

black beans
chick peas
pinto beans
green peas
northern peas
soy beans

FAT BURNING FLAVORING

This is a list of fat burning flavoring that adds flavor without adding fat. Some of these flavorings can be used as topping in place of fat.

Example: Chile Sauce on salad served on top of baked potato.

Some of these flavorings can be used as a substitute for butter.

Example: Clear Seasoned Broth or Horseradish whipped into mashed potatoes

or herbs and/or low sodium soy sauce added to pasta.

Try new ideas and learn to substitute. Have fun with your favorite recipes.

FAT BURNING FOOD WITHOUT ADDING CALORIES BUT PROVIDE FLAVOR

bouillon cubes
chili sauce
clear broth
cocktail sauce
cranberry sauce
fruit spread
herbs
horseradish
ketchup
lemon juice
lime juice
reduced fat mayonnaise
mint sauce
mustards
pickles
salsa
relishes
soy sauce, low sodium
spices
steak sauce
vinegar
worcestershire sauce

SECTION - C

Section-C plays a primary role in showing you how to get rid of some of the old and opening the doors for some of the new. For healthier eating, healthier shopping is the key. You may have to clear out some of the items in your pantry for a fresh start. Most people quickly run out of ideas of what is healthy to eat. This section strongly supports Sections A and B by providing you with even more easy and fun ideas for eating healthier for life. It takes the guesswork out of what you can eat. By the time you complete this section, you will know how to create your own food list and easy meal combination based on your likes and dislikes. It is as easy as your A B C's.

HEALTHY SHOPPING IS THE FIRST STEP. IT IS A MUST FOR HEALTHY WEIGHT LOSS AND MAINTENANCE

Before you can start to lose weight the healthy way, you must have enough of the right foods in your house.

Shopping is the first step for a healthy weight loss and lifetime maintenance. What you already have in your pantry or refrigerator is what you will usually eat. So for this reason you need to read food labels and compare like products before shopping. When trying to reduce total fat, sugar and calories, you will never need to count fat gram or calories if you first start off by shopping right. You don't have to give up the foods yo like. Instead, buy foods that have less fat and sugar more often. There is no need to change your pantry or refrigerator overnight. Add new food gradually over several weeks. You will need this time to test new products. For a healthy weight loss maintenance, you need to buy more lower-fat products and avoid stocking up on concentrated snacks. Read the labels to help you keep more healthy foods on hand at all times.

The best time to grocery shop is after you have eaten. Shopping when you're hungry may lead to what is known as impulse buying, especially junk food.

Make a shopping list. Try to stay with it. This will help you avoid buying unnecessary foods or too much food higher in calorie and fat.

*Manufacturers are coming out with so many lower fat versions from their regular products line which also includes fresh and process meats. Beef and pork are leaner now.

Buying Fat Free – Low Fat products, some are very tasty. These items are good to balance your fat intake by trying to keep the meal in a 35% fat range. Lower fat and no fat are also good for food preparation especially when you may want to reduce the total fat but not cut the fat too low. Some fat is needed too.

Eating more of the right kinds of fat is better. Researchers are taking notice that a fat intake too low does not work. A fat intake lower than 30% or lower as most people are aware, find that the so-called low fat or very low fat diet is too hard to maintain, and that dieters could not stick with it too long. Dieting just does not work. A healthy meal plan is easier and for years I have been recommending to my clients, a fat intake of 35% is better and the results have been good.

Some fats that you were told not to eat on the low fat or very low fat diet, are allowed on a healthy meal plan. They are unsaturated fats, but you still need to control the amount you consume.

- vegetable oils

- nuts and seeds

- olives

- avocado

- mayonnaise

A lower fat shopping guide for the beginner has been provided. This will teach you how to read food labels in order to determine the food portion sizes, fat grams for weight control and maintenance. You will learn how to stock your kitchen so that you can begin to eat healthy without counting calories or fat grams. Start slow, only buy a few new items at a time. If the new food passes your taste test, start making your own healthy shopping list. Use the new shopping list for about a month or so, then start using the more advanced shopping guide list provided. This program will show you how to eat healthier but will not tell you how much or what to eat. When you eat healthier, you should start losing weight without dieting, and you need to eat to lose and maintain the weight lost.

READING FOOD LABELS

A rule of thumb that will help when buying lower fat foods is to look for 3 grams of fat or less per serving. 5 grams of fat is also good depending on the type of food and serving size. If you are buying foods with higher grams of fat per serving, just try to balance higher fat meals with lower fat meals. Eat lower fat more often and enjoy higher fat meals at time.

GROCERY SHOPPING GUIDE (READ THE LABELS) – FAT GRAMS

This shopping guide will also help you read food labels and compare like products. When eating your one or two fatty or sweeter meal for the week, I would want you to buy those items as needed. Do not stock them in your pantry or refrigerator.

LABEL READING

DAIRY

Buy skim milk or 1% low fat cheese with less than 6 grams fat per ounce.

Yogurt with less than 2 grams fat per cup

Light sour cream with less than 2 grams of fat per ounce

BREAD, CEREALS AND GRAINS

With 2 grams fat or less per serving

CRACKERS

4 grams of fat or less

COOKIES

With less than 4 grams fat per ounce

CHIPS

4 grams of fat or less per ounce

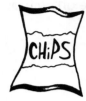

FRUITS AND VEGETABLES

No restrictions

CANNED AND FROZEN FRUITS AND VEGETABLES

Buy those with no added fat or with less sugar

SOUPS

With 2 grams fat or less per serving

LEAN MEAT

Buy more often these cuts

Beef: round, loin, sirloin, chuck arm

Pork: tenderloin, center loin, ham

Veal: all cuts except ground

Lamb: leg, loin, fore shanks

Poultry: Buy ground chicken or turkey that is 91%-99% fat free, buy

Light meat without the skin more often. May buy poultry with skin and remove

more often after cooking before eating.

LUNCH MEATS

Choose those with less than 4 grams fat per ounce

FROZEN ENTREES

Buy those with 9 grams fat per serving or less

FATS

- Margarine: choose reduced fat or those in tub

- Oils: canola, olive oil, corn, sunflower, safflower

- Mayonnaise and salad dressings: serve smaller portions or buy reduced-fat type

- Nuts: use in moderation as a snack or mixed with salads, fruits, vegetables, etc.

LOWER FAT SHOPPING FOR THE BEGINNER

HIGHER IN FAT AND CALORIES	FAT GRAMS	LOWER IN FAT	FAT GRAMS
Whole milk 8 oz.	8.9	Skim milk 8 oz. Milk 2% 8 oz. Milk 1% 8 oz.	0 0.5 0.3
Buttermilk 4 oz.	1.1	Low fat buttermilk 4 oz.	1
Evaporated milk 4 oz.	19	Evaporated skim milk 4 oz.	1
Milk chocolate 1 oz.	9	Licorice 1 oz. Hot cocoa mix w/water (1 pk)	0 1
Whole plain yogurt 8 oz.	7.4	Plain nonfat yogurt 8 oz.	3
Ricotta cheese 4 oz.	16	Ricotta part-skim 4 oz.	9.8
Regular cottage cheese 4 oz.	5	Low fat cottage cheese 4 oz.	1.2
Sour cream ¼ cup	9	Reduced fat sour cream ¼ cup	4
Cream cheese 1 oz.	9.9	Lite cream cheese 1 oz.	4.7
American cheese 1 oz.	7	Low fat American cheese 1 oz.	4.3
Swiss cheese 1 oz.	6.8	Low fat Swiss cheese 1 oz.	3.7
Cheddar cheese 1 oz.	9	Reduced fat Cheddar 1 oz.	5
Mozzarella cheese 1 oz.	6.1	Part skim mozzarella 1 oz.	3.7
Grated parmesan cheese 1 oz.	9	Hoop cheese 1 oz.	Trace
Butter 1 tablespoon	12	Whipped butter 1 tablespoon Butter spray Butter flavored granules	9.2 0 0
Margarine 1 tablespoon	12	Reduced fat margarine 1 tablespoon Vegetable 1 tablespoon Vegetable cooking spray 1 tablespoon	6 4 1
Mayonnaise 1 tablespoon	11.2	Reduced fat mayonnaise 1 tablespoon	2.9
Salad dressing 1 tablespoon	7	Salad dressing reduced fat 1	0

		tablespoon	
		Homemade salad dressing 1 tablespoon	0
Peanut butter 1 tablespoon	8.2	Peanut butter reduced fat	0
HIGHER IN FAT AND CALORIES	**FAT GRAMS**	**LOWER IN FAT**	**FAT GRAMS**
Whole egg 1 large	5	Egg white, 2 large	1
		Egg substitute	0
Croissant (1)	12	Raisin toast w/fruit spread	2
Fruit danish (1)	14	Bagel with fruit spread	3
Bagel with butter (1)	15	Bagel with fruit spread	3
Apple turnover (1)	17	Crumb cake	4
French toast (1 slice)	6.7	French toast w/skim milk (1 slice)	5
		Reduced fat pancake mix 4	1.9
Caramel bar cookies (2)	16	Oatmeal cookie (1)	6
Chocolate chip cookies (2)	10	Fig bars (2)	2
		Cream filled cookies (2)	4
		Graham crackers (2)	1
		Vanilla wafers (7)	7
		Ginger snap cookies (3)	2
		Angel food cake (1 slice)	0.1
Ice cream – vanilla (1/2 cup)	14.3	Low fat ice cream vanilla (1/2 cup)	4
		Frozen juice bar (1)	0
		Frozen low fat yogurt 8 oz.	3.5
		Sorbet dessert (1/2 cup)	0
Potato chips 1 oz.	10.1	Fat free potato chips 1 oz.	0
		Pretzels 1 oz.	1
		Popcorn air popped	0.3
		Low fat tortilla chips ¾ oz.	0.5
Vanilla pudding 1 cup	8	Vanilla pudding w/low fat milk 1 cup	3
		Vanilla pudding w/skim milk 1 cup	0
		Chocolate pudding w/skim milk 1 cup	0
		Gelatin dessert 1 cup	0
Short ribs 3 oz.	36	Sirloin steak trim 3 oz.	15
Brisket of beef 3 oz.	27.8	Roast beef, round tip 3 oz.	15.3
Pork spare ribs 3 oz.	27	Pork fresh loin, lean 3 oz.	4.2
Lamb shoulder little fat 3 oz.	20.9	Lamb shoulder lean 3 oz.	8
Lamb chop loin 2.5 oz.	20.9	Leg of lamb, lean 3 oz.	6
Chicken w/skin light 3.5 oz.	10.9	Chicken without skin light 3.5 oz.	4.5
Chicken with skin dark 3.5 oz.	15.8	Chicken without skin dark	9.7

		3.5 oz.	
Turkey with skin white 3.5 oz.	8.3	Turkey without skin white 3.5	3.2
Turkey with skin dark 3.5 oz	11.5	Turkey without skin dark 3.5	7.2
Veal rib roast 3 oz.	14.4	Veal cutlet broiled 3 oz.	9.1
HIGHER IN FAT AND CALORIES	**FAT GRAMS**	**LOWER IN FAT**	**FAT GRAMS**
Veal parmagiana 4.2 oz.	18	Veal loin lean 3 oz.	3
		Veal ground lean 4 oz.	6
Pastrami, beef 2 oz.	16.6	Pastrami, turkey 2 oz.	7
Knockwurst (1)	18.9	Turkey frank (1)	3
Bologna 2 oz.	16	Bologna, lean 2 oz.	2
Pork breakfast sausage 1 oz.	7	Turkey breakfast sausage 1 oz.	2
Fried shrimp 3 oz.	10.4	Shrimp broiled 3 oz.	0.9
Tuna in oil, drained 3 oz.	7	Tuna in water 3 oz.	0.5
		Lobster, broiled 3 oz.	0.5
		Crab cake (1)	5
Bacon 2-3 thin slices	7-10	Canadian bacon 2 slices 2 oz.	4
		Turkey bacon 2 slices	5
		Extra lean ham 2 oz.	1.5
		Extra lean turkey bacon 2 slices	1.5
		Fresh turkey bacon 2 slices	0
Creamed herring ¼ cup	7	Uncreamed herring ¼ cup	5
Potato nuggets frozen 8 oz.	14	Baked potato with skin (1 Med)	0.2
Hash browns ½ cup	10.9	Mashed potato with low fat milk ½ cup	1.5

SHOPPING FOR HEALTHY DESSERTS

LOWER CALORIE DESSERTS:

- ▢ Fresh sliced strawberries, blueberries, or raspberries, and about 1 tablespoon of cold water and 1 teaspoon of sugar. Chill and serve over a slice of angel food cake.

- ▢ Small amount of raisin and nuts mixed with plain vanilla flavored low-fat yogurt

- ▢ Homemade bread pudding made with skim milk or 1% milk, and raisins or canned fruit cocktail, vanilla flavoring, nutmeg or cinnamon, egg white, and reduce the amount of sugar (no butter – bake)

- ▢ Plain regular Jell-O with Cool Whip, fat-free topping

- ☐ Fruited Jell-O with Cool Whip, fat-free topping (fruit cocktail canned in natural juice)

- ☐ Fruited Jell-O with sliced canned peaches or pears

- ☐ Fruited Jell-O with canned peach or pear halves (lay fruit out in a square dish, pour Jell-O over fruit, let gel, slice in squares, top with Cool Whip fat-free topping with a ¼ cup maraschino cherries

- ☐ Fruited Jell-O with sliced fresh bananas, let gel

- ☐ Jell-O instant pudding made with skim milk or 1% milk

- ☐ Banana pudding made with vanilla instant pudding mix, made with skim milk, layer with fresh sliced bananas and vanilla wafer (follow direction of package using skim milk or 1% fat milk) and add less waffles.

- ☐ Jell-O instant pudding made with skim milk mix in drained canned fruit cocktail or peaches, natural juice or light syrup; chill.

- ☐ Ginger snaps and reduced fat milk or hot tea.

- ☐ Fresh fruit

- ☐ Diced cut-up canned pineapples, natural juice, topped with Cool Whip Fat-Free, or topped with Jell-O Instant Pudding made with skim milk, or 1% milk, sprinkled with crushed nuts (small amount).

Advanced Shopping List

WEIGHT MAINTENANCE AND LOSS – ADVANCED MEAT SHOPPING GUIDE

Eat more very lean, and medium fat meats. Eat high fat meat no more than once a week or save that high fat meat for that special occasion, e.g., birthday party, family cookout, etc. If you eat high fat for a meal or for that day, it is the total fat intake for the week that counts. If you eat high fat meat, have as much of the visible fat removed before cooking.

- Meats are grouped according to fat contents. In order to lose and maintain your weight, you need to eat leaner cuts of meat and poultry

- There are 4 groups of meat, high fat meat has been omitted:

  1. **Very lean group** – eat more

  2. **Lean group** – eat more

  3. **Medium fat group** – eat in moderation

To help maintain your weight, eat more from groups 1 and 2.

MEAT GROUPING:

GROUP 1. VERY LEAN MEAT (EAT MORE):

- Laura's Lean Beef
- Chicken, white meat (no skin)
- Turkey, white meat (no skin)
- Cornish hen (no skin)

- Duck (no skin)
- Pheasant (no skin)
- Ostrich
- Buffalo

GROUP 2. LEAN MEAT (EAT MORE): TRIM FAT

LEAN BEEF:

- ☐ Top round
- ☐ Bottom round
- ☐ Flank steak
- ☐ Sirloin
- ☐ Tenderloin
- ☐ Chuck steak
- ☐ Chuck roast
- ☐ Rib roast
- ☐ Rib rump
- ☐ T-bone steak
- ☐ Cubed steak
- ☐ Porterhouse
- ☐ Lean ground round

LEAN POULTRY:

- ☐ Chicken dark meat (no skin)
- ☐ Turkey dark meat (no skin)
- ☐ Duck (no skin)
- ☐ Goose (no skin, drain off fat)
- ☐ Rabbit (no skin)
- ☐ Processed meat (2 grams or less fat)
- ☐ Reduced fat hotdogs (3 grams or less fat)

LEAN PORK:

- Lean fresh ham
- Lean boiled ham
- Lean canned ham
- Lean cured ham
- Tenderloin cuts
- Center loin chop
- Canadian bacon

LEAN LAMB:

- Lamb roast
- Lamb chop
- Lamb leg

LEAN VEAL:

- Lean veal chop
- Veal roast (trim)

GROUP 3.   MEDIUM FAT MEAT (EAT LESS): In Moderation (TRIM OFF FAT)

MEDIUM FAT BEEF:

- Prime rib
- Prime cuts of steak
- Ground beef
- Short ribs
- Corned beef

MEDIUM FAT PORK:

- Pork chops, trim fat
- Top loin
- Cutlet
- Boston butt
- Sausage, with 4-5 grams of fat per ounce

MEDIUM FAT LAMB:

- Rib roast
- Ground lamb

MEDIUM FAT VEAL:

- Ground veal
- Cutlet
- Cubed

MEDIUM FAT POULTRY:

- Chicken with skin
- Turkey with skin

FISH LIST – EAT ANY KIND OF FISH:

- Clams
- Crab
- Lobster
- Scallops
- Shrimp
- Imitation shellfish
- Cod

- Flounder
- Haddock
- Halibut
- Trout
- Tuna (fresh or canned in water)
- Herring
- Oyster

- ☐   Salmon   •   Plus others

Try to eat fish 2 or 3 times a week.

CHEESE:

COTTAGE CHEESE:

- ☐   Creamed cottage cheese, less fat

- ☐   Cottage cheese fat free

- ☐   Cottage cheese, 4% milk

RICOTTA CHEESE:

- ☐   Ricotta, lite

- ☐   Ricotta, skim

- ☐   Ricotta, fat free

OTHER CHEESES: (FAT FREE, PART SKIM, 2% MILK)

- ☐   American

- ☐   Cheddar

- ☐   Mozzarella

- ☐   Swiss (etc.)

EGGS:

- ☐   Eggs, fresh, Limit to 3 per week

- ☐   Egg substitute with 55-80 calories per serving

TOFU

MILK AND YOGURT:

- ☐   Low Fat Milk

-     Skim Milk

- ☐ 1% Milk

- ☐ Dry non fat milk

- ☐ Buttermilk, low fat, non fat

- ☐ Evaporated, Skim or fat free

- ☐ Sweet acidophilus milk

- ☐ Yogurt plain, low fat, fat free

- ☐ Yogurt fruit flavored, non fat, or low fat

OTHER:

- ☐ Creamers, nondairy, liquid

- ☐ Creamers, nondairy, powdered

BREADS AND STARCHS (Also use complex carbohydrates list high in fiber on page)

BREADS:

- ☐ Bagel

- ☐ Biscuit, homemade, reduced fat mix

- ☐ Bun, hamburger or hot dog

- ☐ Cornbread, homemade

- ☐ Raisin, unfrosted

- • Pancake, low fat mix

- • Pita bread

- • Rye, pumpernickel

- • Tortilla, 6 in. across

BREADS: (continued)

- ☐ English muffins

- ☐ Muffin, homemade

- ☐ Poultry stuffing

- ☐ Plain roll

- • Whole wheat

- • White (including French, Italian)

- • Tortilla, flour or corn

- • Waffle, low fat mix

- ☐ Roll, hard

CRACKERS:

- ☐ Breadsticks
- ☐ Graham crackers
- ☐ Matzo
- ☐ Meal-mates sesame bread wafers
- ☐ Melba toast
- ☐ Rye krisp
- ☐ Saltines
- ☐ Wheat thins

- Biscuits
- Wheatsworth
- Oyster crackers
- Pretzels
- Dutch
- Sticks
- Large rings

CEREALS:

- ☐ Bran cereal, shredded & bud types
- ☐ Flaked cereal
- ☐ Grits
- ☐ Hot cereal (oatmeal, cream of wheat)
- ☐ Puffed cereal

PASTA: (cooked)

- Egg noodles
- Lasagna noodles
- Macaroni
- Spaghetti
- Chowmein noodles, thin

RICE:

- ☐ Brown rice
- ☐ Long grain, enriched rice
- ☐ Rice-a-Roni, homemade
- ☐ Rice pilaf

FLOUR AND MEAL:

- Barley, dry
- Bread crumbs
- Cornflakes crumbs
- Cornstarch
- ☐ Cornmeal
- ☐ Flour

BEANS: (cooked)

- ☐ Limas
- ☐ White
- ☐ Pinto
- ☐ Kidney
- ☐ Navy

- Garbanzo beans
- Chick peas
- Baked beans
- Lentils
- etc.

PEAS:

- ☐ Green
- ☐ Sweet
- ☐ Black-eyed or cow peas
- ☐ Split

CORN:

- Ear
- Kernels or cream style
- Popcorn (air popped) (no butter added)

POTATOES:

- ☐ White
- ☐ Baking
- ☐ Sweet potato, yams

OTHER:

- Parsnips
- Pumpkin, winter squash
- Mixed vegetables
- ☐ Tomato puree/paste

VEGETABLES:

- ☐ Artichoke
- ☐ Asparagus
- ☐ Beans (green, wax, Italian)
- ☐ Bean sprouts
- ☐ Beets

- Mushrooms
- Napolitos
- Okra
- Onions
- Pea Pods

• ☐ Broccoli	• Pepper, bell
• ☐ Brussel sprouts	• Pimento
• ☐ Cabbage (cooked)	• Radishes
• ☐ Carrots	• Rutabaga
• ☐ Cauliflower	• Sauerkraut
• ☐ Celery	• Shallots
• ☐ Chicory	• Spinach
• ☐ Cucumbers	• Sprouts (alfalfa and bean)
• ☐ Escarole	• Tomatoes
• ☐ Eggplant	• Turnips
• ☐ Greens (all kinds)	• Watercress
• ☐ Jicama	• Waterchestnuts
• ☐ Kohlrabi	• Yellow squash
• ☐ Leeks	• Zucchini
• ☐ Lettuce	• Tomato Juice, vegetable juice cocktail

*Avoid breaded fried vegetables, vegetable seasoned with bacon fat, salt pork or vegetables in cream or cheese sauces.

Ex:　1)　Bacon fat, salt pork – use smoke turkey (no skin) or Canadian Bacon.

　　　2)　Cream Sauce – use 1% milk or fat-free evaporated milk.

FRUIT HEALTHY SHOPPING GUIDE:

FRESH, FROZEN, AND UNSWEETENED CANNED FRUIT

• Apple	• Mango
• Applesauce (unsweetened)	• Nectarine

- Apricots
- Banana
- Blackberries
- Blueberries
- Cantaloupe
- Cherries (canned)
- Figs
- Fruit Cocktail
- Grapefruit
- Grapefruit (segments)
- Grapes
- Honeydew Melon
- Kiwi
- Mandarin Oranges

- Orange
- Papaya
- Peach
- Pear
- Pears (canned)
- Persimmon (native)
- Pineapple
- Plum (raw)
- Pomegranate
- Raspberries
- Strawberries
- Tangerine
- Watermelon

DRIED FRUIT:

- ☐ Apples
- ☐ Apricots
- ☐ Dates
- ☐ Figs
- ☐ Prunes
- ☐ Raisins

FRUIT JUICE:

- Apple juice/cider
- Cranberry juice cocktail
- Grape juice
- Orange juice
- Pineapple juice
- Prune juice

HEALTHY SOUP/CANNED (Some reduced fat canned soup may be higher in sodium)

Check healthy food store for healthy soup low in fat, calories and sodium.

Clear broth with diced chicken.

Clear Chicken broth with white rice.

Broth with onion

Light Minestrone Soup

Light tomato soup

Light vegetable soup

Light bean soup

Light split pea soup with diced Canadian bacon, plus more

These soups can also be made homemade reduced fat.

THE FOLLOWING ARE UNSATURATED FATS WHICH ARE GOOD IF USED IN

MODERATION:

Nuts: almonds
brazil nuts
cashews
chestnuts
coconut (unsweetened)
filberts or hazel nuts
hickory nuts
macadamias
peanuts
pecans
pine nuts
pistachios
pumpkin seeds
soy nuts, toasted
sunflower seeds
walnuts

Oil: corn
cottonseed
safflower
soybean
sunflower
olive
peanut

Salad Dressing and Spread:

Regular mayonnaise, smaller amount
Mayonnaise, reduced calories, fat free
Salad Dressing, reduced calorie, fat free

*IN PLACE OF REGULAR BUTTER AND MARGARINE:

Whipped Butter
Trans-fatty Acid free (the best)

FAT FREE FOODS – LITTLE OR NO CALORIES

There are a limited amount of foods with so little calories that can be consumed

as desired. Use the following list or groups of listings as a guide. Many on the free items provided are herbs and spices, which add flavor to other foods. Many of these foods can also be eaten along with other food to save on calories and will help fill you up. Some of them make good snacks between meals and will help prevent hunger. Example: 1-cup hot clear consommé with 2 tablespoons of cooked rice and two crackers.

FREE CALORIES OR VERY LOW:

DRINKS – FREE

Water
Carbonated drinks – sugar free
Carbonated water
Club soda
Cocoa powder, (unsweetened)
Postum
Tonic water
Coffee, Tea

FREE VEGETABLE:

Raw vegetable, 1 cup
Cabbage
Celery
Chinese cabbage
Cucumber
Green onion
Hot peppers
Mushrooms
Radishes
Zucchini

CONDIMENTS FREE:

Catsup (1 tbsp)
Horseradish
Mustard
Pickles, dill or sour
Taco sauce (1 tbsp)
Vinegar

SOUP-FREE

Bouillon fat free
Consommé clear
Fat free

FRUIT-FREE

Cranberries (unsweetened ½ cup)
Rhubarb (unsweetened)

COOKING OIL – FREE:

Non stick pan spray

FREE BUTTER

Butter buds
Butter Flavoring
Non-stick, butter flavor spray
Butter spray

EACH DAY ONLY:

Cocktail Sauce – 1 tbsp
Chili Sauce – 1 tbsp
Salsa, free or reduced

SEASONINGS – FREE:

Basil (fresh)
Celery seeds
Cinnamon
Chili powder
Chives
Curry
Dill
Flavoring extracts:
Vanilla, almond, walnut
Peppermint, lemon
Butter flavoring
Garlic
Garlic powder
Herbs
Hot pepper sauce
Lemon

Lemon juice
Lemon pepper
Lime
Lime juice
Mint
Onion powder
Oregano
Paprika
Pepper
Pimento
Spices
Soy Sauce
Soy Sauce, low sodium
Soy Sauce, "lite"
Wine, used in cooking (1/4 cup)
Worcester shire sauce

SHOPPING GUIDE

YOU DO NOT NEED TO FOLLOW A MEAL PLAN, JUST EAT SMART

If you shop high fat, you will eat high fat.

DRESSING UP LOW CALORIE FOODS

Eating lower fat food is good, but the dressing you put on the food you eat can get you into trouble.

Baked potatoes – a healthy low-fat food

	HIGHER FAT	**LOWER FAT**
Baked potatoes	1. Sour Cream	Reduced fat sour cream
		Reduced fat yogurt
	2. Butter	Trans fat free (buttery spread)
		Salsa
	3. Regular Cheese	Reduced fat cheese
		½ portion regular cheese

with veggies

sprinkle with small amount of

cheese

HEALTHY TOPPINGS FOR BAGELS, CRACKERS, RICE CAKES, ETC.

The average American uses too much butter.

- Spread with smaller amount of jelly or jam

- Spread with natural fruit spread

- Spread with reduced fat or no fat cream cheese

- Top with reduced fat cheese

- Spread with reduced fat cottage cheese mixed with natural fruit spread

- Top with seafood cocktail sauce

- Top with salsa

- Top with chili sauce

- Top with seasoned sliced ham, turkey, or chicken breast (teriyaki sauce, sweet and sour sauce, lemon and pepper sauce, mustard sauce etc.)

- Spread with reduced fat or non-fat cream cheese mixed with raisin or shredded carrots mixture or both.

- Spread with reduced fat or non-fat cream cheese and chives mixture.

- Top with small amount tuna salad mixture, reduced fat mayonnaise or homemade mayonnaise or less regular mayonnaise.

- Spread whole cranberry sauce on top of thin slice white turkey meat breast and serve on crackers, toast or bagel.

- Spread on low-fat bean dip.

- Spread on reduced fat peanut butter or reduced fat peanut butter with fruit spread.

- Rice cake with banana slices.

- Reduced fat soft cheese mix with pureed fruits, spread on whole-wheat toast or saltine type of crackers.

- Low fat soft cheese mixed with small amount of honey, spread on wheat crackers or bagels.

- Low fat cheese mixed with fruit spreads.

SHOPPING GUIDE

HEALTHY SALSA – Keep this in the house. This makes a healthy convenient snack and can be used to dress up a main meal.

LOWER FAT EATING – LOW FAT SALSA

COMMERCIAL MARINARA SAUCES (Be creative)

Salsa has many uses. It adds flavor without adding fat and can be used as a healthy snack or with a main meal.

- Take your favorite marinara sauce, stir in a few tablespoons prepared pesto and add to pasta.

- For a nice western omelet, sauce

  1 fresh chopped zucchini, ¼ pound chopped mushrooms, and 1 small chopped or sliced onion into mixture 3 to 4 tablespoons of marinara sauce. (Will make enough sauce for four omelets).

- Turkey loaf, cover with marinara sauce at the last half hour of baking.

- Lean chopped beef sautéed, drain off fat. Toss in cooked pasta and enough commercial marinara sauce, heat and serve. Make your own healthy hamburger helper with salsa.

- Lean hamburger or turkey burger on a bun, topped with sliced onion and commercial marinara sauce.

- Turkey sandwich, spread with a mixture of 2 parts reduced fat mayonnaise with 1 part salsa.

- Bacon, lettuce and tomato sandwich (BLT)

  In Place of regular bacon use Canadian bacon, topped with your favorite tomato salsa, or use 3 slices of regular thin bacon, grill on rack to let grease drain off.

- Grilled fish (tuna, salmon, swordfish), top with salsa, chopped onions or chopped cilantro.

- Salsa chili – 1 pound of ground turkey, 1 small chopped onions, 2 cloves fresh crushed garlic, 2 teaspoons chili powder, sautéed, then stir in 1 can kidney beans (DO NOT DRAIN) and 1 cup of tomato base salsa, heat and serve over rice.

- Shrimp with salsa, stir fry 1 medium sliced green and red pepper, 1 small sliced onion, 2 cloves crushed garlic or garlic powder to taste, use small amount of olive oil or vegetable cooking spray, cook slightly. Add 1 pound cleaned and washed shrimp, let cook for about 4 minutes, and then stir in 1 ½ cup of salsa, bring to a slight boil. Serve over steamed rice or pasta. Serves 6.

- Mexican corn, sauté 1 small diced onion, 2 chopped medium zucchini with a small amount of vegetable oil. Then add 2 cups of frozen whole kernel corn or 1 can drained corn, 1 cup salsa, simmer 1 minute, serve as a side dish or as a main vegetable dish serve over rice or noodles.

- Omelet, use one egg yolk to two egg whites per person. Sauté sliced green pepper, sliced onions, mix with salsa, set aside. Beat eggs with salt, pepper to taste with a small amount of water. Spray pan with vegetable cooking spray, cook egg mixture on both sides, then place salsa mixture on one side of omelet and fold. Make one omelet at a time.

- Reduced fat salsa dip, 1 can of drained black beans pureed, then stir in 1 ½ cups of your favorite tomato base salsa.

- Mexican scramble eggs, 2 egg whites to 1 egg yolk per person. Mix in 2 teaspoon of chopped chilies (jar) and 2 teaspoon tomato salsa scramble and serve over toast.

- Mexican corn bread – (10 ounces) box of corn bread, follow direction of package. Mix together 1 can whole kernel corn, drain ½ cup chopped chilies, ½ cup drained salsa. Add to corn mixture and bake.

SHOPPING GUIDE

If you shop healthy, you will eat healthy – SALADS GUIDE

Many people believe that the word salad means healthy. Some salads are loaded with fat and sugar and are high in calories. Use this list as a guide when shopping for salad and salad dressing.

COMBINATIONS:

- Cucumber thin sliced – vinegar marinade

- Cucumber and onion – low fat sour cream dressing 2% or vinegar oil marinade, use less oil

- Cucumber slices and tomato slices – French or Russian dressing marinade, 2% or non fat

- Tomatoes Oreganata – tomato slices or wedges, oregano, salt, red onion slices, small amount of oil and vinegar for marinade

FROZEN VEGETABLES (Slightly cook and chilled)

1. Mixed vegetable salad, add chopped celery, reduced fat mayo, or half regular mayo with plain yogurt.

2. Brussel sprouts – carrots thin slices – marinade vinegar oil marinade

3. Broccoli vinegrette – vinegar oil, use less oil. Garnish with ½ boiled chopped egg per serving.

4. Snow pea pods – alone or combination with bean sprouts.

5. Italian green beans with diced tomatoes, shredded carrot, diced onion.

6. Black-eye pea salad with chopped celery, and onion, oil and vinegar, or mix with healthy tomato salsa.

7. Wax beans with sliced tomatoes and diced onion

8. Whole green beans with pimentos.

Note: Be creative when shopping for salad dressing and toppings. There are many lower fat, non-fat dressing in the market. Lower fat items have improved in taste.

BEET SALADS:

1. Sliced beets pickled with onion sliced

2. Small whole beets (cans) diced onions

3. Julienne beets (cans) pickled or sour cream, with reduced fat sour cream or homemade sour cream

BEAN SALADS:

1. 3 Bean   a) green beans

                 b) kidney bean

                 c) garbanzos

2. Green beans and canned mushroom pieces – diced pimento

3. Wax beans with celery, chopped hard cooked egg

4. Green beans, canned whole corn, sliced ripe olives, diced pimento

COLE SLAW: (with reduced fat dressing)

1. Red and green cabbage cole slaw

2. Cole slaw with pineapple tidbits

3. Cole slaw with caraway seeds

4. Cole slaw with raisins

5.   Cole slaw with pineapple and raisins

6.   Cole slaw with pineapple, raisins and walnuts

CARROTS – SALAD:

1.   Carrot and raisin

2.   Carrot and pineapple and celery (chop)

POTATO SALAD:

1.   Potato salad, reduced fat mayonnaise or small amount of regular mayonnaise with raisins.

2.   Potato salad with eggs (2 white to 1 yolk).

3.   Potato salad with eggs, reduced fat mayonnaise and a teaspoon or two of light mustard for potato salad with slightly cooked chilled mixed vegetable.

MACARONI OR OTHER PASTA:

1.   Pasta and tuna, reduced fat mayonnaise with mustard or smaller amount of regular mayo

2.   Pasta with shredded carrot and diced tomato, vinegar marinade, or reduced fat mayonnaise or small amount of regular mayo.

3.   Curry mayonnaise with macaroni, diced turkey (white meat), chopped celery, raisins and nuts (or add curry powder to home-made reduced fat mayonnaise)

4.   Pasta with chilled mixed vegetable with healthy dressing.

5.   Pasta with diced hard-boiled egg, relish and reduced fat mayonnaise or vinegar oil marinade.

SHOPPING GUIDE – GOOD FOR MAIN MEAL, DESSERT OR SNACK

FRUIT SALAD – COMBINATION IN NATURAL JUICE, DRAINED

Combine: Orange sections

Grapefruit sections

Banana slices

Mandarin orange

FROZEN FRUITS:

Combine: Bing cherries

Pear slices

Peach slices

CANNED FRUITS:

Combine: Pineapple slices

Peach halves

Pear halves

MELON SLICES – OR DICED:

Combine: Cantaloupe

Honeydew

Watermelon

Etc.

SHOPPING IDEAS FOR SNACKING:

HEALTHY DIPPERS can be eaten in place of higher fat snacks. Stay away from the traditional dippers like potato chips and corn dips or high fat crackers.

TRY THESE HEALTHY DIPPERS:

VEGETABLE DIPPERS:

Broccoli, cauliflower, carrots, bell peppers, zucchini, yellow squash, eggplant, celery, tomatoes, steam whole green beans, cucumber, baby corn.

STARCH DIPPERS:

Saltines, reduced fat potatoes or corn chips, pretzels, rice crackers, rye crisps, wheat snacks crackers, reduced fat sweet potato chips, reduced fat crackers.

FRUIT DIPPERS (sliced, diced, cubed)

Sliced apples, pears, peaches, nectarines, strawberries, melons, dried fruits, and pineapples.

Reduced fat dips recipes for the low fat dippers are provided in Section D.

SECTION-D

You cannot get too much of good healthy information; more is better. Enjoy eating healthier without giving up taste. Yes, you can have your cake and eat it too. There is no need to count calories or fat grams. This is not a recipe book, but this Section will show you how you can still eat many of your loved foods. I have provided some recipe makeovers and other tips for easy, lower fat cooking. When you shop right, you must also cook right to control total fat and sugar intake to avoid unwanted weight gain and more. This section is like putting the icing on the cake. A healthy salad needs a healthy dressing or it can easily be taken out of the healthy range. Many people take a healthy dish and load it up with unhealthy toppings.

Enjoy eating healthier without giving up taste.

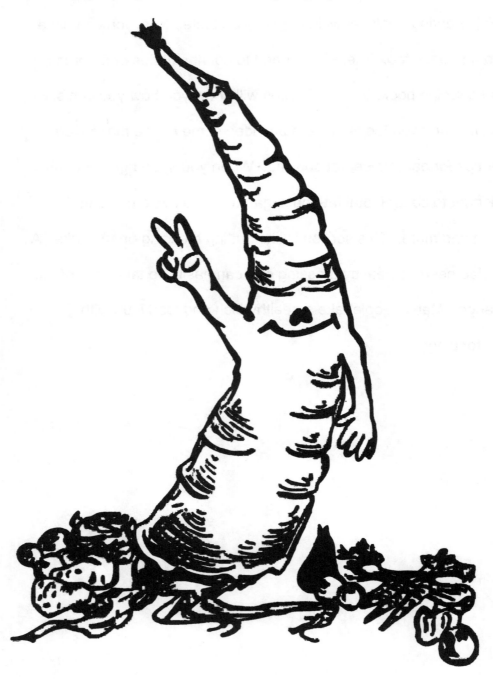

LOWER FAT COOKING/EATING

You must control total fat and sugar too when cooking and eating. Eating healthy for life most of the time is a must for weight loss and maintenance. Eating more good fat and less saturated fat, less total calories, and more fiber and drinking water is the key. You must eat to lose weight.

CUTTING THE FAT - LOWER FAT COOKING IS A MUST

You do not need to give up your favorite foods by eating only healthy food that may be boring to you. You will not remain on a healthy eating plan for long if you are eating foods you do not like.

Eat your favorite high fat foods about two times a week. Also, find out how you can get these foods in a lower-fat version that tastes good to you and or other substitutes without added fat and sugar. Learn how to prepare some of these foods yourself.

Lower-fat cooking and meal preparation can bring down your daily fat intake within a healthy range.

The easiest way to control what goes into your food is by preparing your meal at home. Use as many lower fat products or ingredients as possible. Follow the low fat healthy shopping tips provided. Use these items in your food preparation at home. Do not add unnecessary fats or sugar in the preparation of your meal. Learn how to substitute high fat for low fat ingredients in cooking.

If you do not follow the lower fat shopping and cooking tips, you can very easily take a meal out of the control healthy fat intake range of 30 to 35%.

LEAN MEAT – FOR CONTROLLING FAT AND TOTAL CALORIES

There are newer lean cuts of meat that make low fat cooking easy. At one time, chicken breast skinless was known as the only healthy low fat meat. Today, you can get leaner cuts of beef and pork that come close in fat content to skinless cooked chicken breast, which contains just 3 grams of fat per 3-ounce serving. Beef tenderloin comes in close at 4 grams of fat per 3-ounce serving. The cholesterol contents of chicken, beef, and pork is about the same, which ranges between 20 to 25 milligrams per ounce.

Other low fat meats are on the rise. Buffalo, Venison, Elk, and Ostrich are low in fat and contain about as much protein and as many vitamins and minerals as domesticated meats.

If lean meat is not cooked properly, it will get tough.

LEAN MEAT COOKING TIPS:

- Use very little salt with lean meat cooking. Too much salt may toughen meat during cooking, but a small amount of salt should not hurt and will provide flavor.

- When marinating lean cuts of meat, do not keep too long in a high acidic marinade; it will become tough.

- Cook lean meat quickly. Cooking for long periods of time, especially steaks will become tough. Lower fat steak or roast should be cooked at a high temperature.

- When braising or stewing lean meat, use low heat.

- To provide flavor to lean meat, sauté onions, bell peppers, chilies, or other spices. Add to an oil-based mixture and marinade the meat.

TRIM THE FAT

Trim off the fat from meats like steaks, pork chops, roast beef, etc. before cooking. This may reduce the fat from the meal plan or recipes up to 40% or more.

Chicken prep, you can remove the fat, this may cut the fat from about 50% to 60%. This is good for mix dishes. For baked, broil, grilled chicken if you feel that you want to cook the chicken with the skin on to maintain the flavor, you can just remove the skin after cooking. Not much fat will be absorbed through the chicken but you should discard the drippings.

If you boil the chicken with the skin on, before adding vegetable or thickening agent to the stock, you can remove the skin and also chill stock and skim off the fat. So you see there is no need to count the calories or fat grams.

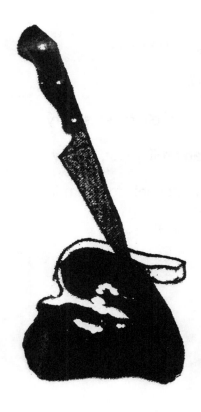

LEAN BEEF COOKING GUIDE

LEAN BEEF - (This group it is best to use dry heat cooking – trim off fat after cooking)

SIRLOIN – Broil, grill, pan broil, roast, stir-fry

TOP LOIN – Broil, grill, pan broil, roast, stir-fry

TENDERLOIN – Broil, grill, pan broil, roast, stir-fry

FLANK – Broil, grill, pan broil, roast, stir-fry

GROUND BEEF (80%, 85%, 90%, 95%) Lean

(Trim off fat before grounding)

GROUND SIRLOIN – Broil, grill, pan broil, roast, stir-fry

GROUND ROUND – Broil, grill, pan broil, roast, stir-fry

LEAN BEEF – (Best to use moist heat cooking – trim fat before cooking)

EYE ROUND – Braise, poach, steam, stew

TOP ROUND – Braise, stew

ROUND TIP – Braise, stew

BOTTOM ROUND – Braise, stew

TENDERLOIN – Poach

LEAN PORK: THE NEW WHITE MEAT

White meat chicken is used a lot in low fat cooking but lean pork is on the rise and is known as the new white meat. Lean pork is 50% leaner than ever. Pork is available in more than 30 different cuts, roasts, steaks, ribs, chops, cubes, and tenderloins, and is adaptable to many different flavors and cooking methods.

Pork cuts are also available pre-trimmed, portioned packaged, lean meat ready to be used as a low fat meat alternative.

Lean cooking is on the rise. Lean pork can be used to prepare and add flavor to Chinese dishes. Use boneless pork tenderloin cuts into strips, stir-fry the strips and toss with a soy-sesame combination and serve over pasta or steamed rice.

For the southwestern cooking, toss lean cooked pork with kidney beans, ripe black olives, green peppers, tomatoes and cumin-oregano spice mixture.

For the healthy cooking craze, pork tenderloins can be sautéed, braised, grilled, stir-fried or roasted. Lean pork can be used in many dishes. Look for healthy recipes, there are many. For a tenderer product, only cook pork to an internal temperature of 145°F to 160°F, which is a big change from the old recommendation of cooking to 185°F. When pork had 50% more fat, it needed to be cooked to a higher temperature to kill harmful bacteria.

LEAN PORK COOKING GUIDE

LEAN PORK (FOR THIS GROUP IT IS BEST TO USE DRY HEAT COOKING, TRIM OFF FAT AFTER COOKING)

PORK TENDERLOIN – Broil, grill, pan broil, roast, stir-fry

LOIN STRIPS – Stir-fry

BONELESS TOP LOIN – Roast, broil, grill, and roast

LOIN CHOP – Broil, grill, pan broil

RIB CHOP – Broil, grill, pan broil

BONELESS RIB ROAST – Grill, roast

BONELESS SIRLOIN CHOP – Broil, grill, pan broil

BONELESS HAM – Broil, grill, pan broil, roast, stir-fry

GROUND PORK VERY LEAN – Broil, grill, pan broil, roast

LEAN PORK (BEST TO USE MOIST HEAT COOKING – TRIM FAT)

LOIN CHOP – Braise

RIB CHOP – Braise

BONELESS SIRLOIN CHOP – Braise

BONELESS RIB ROAST – Braise, stew

TURKEY – FOR CUTTING FAT AND TOTAL CALORIES

Turkey burgers are becoming more popular. It is becoming a common substitute for ground beef and pork. Turkey is lean. A 3-ounce portion has 120 calories, 1 gram of fat and 55 mg of cholesterol.

Make turkey burgers using white meat only. Turkey has a light, milk taste that comes across on its own. Be creative and use it in some of your present beef recipes. Turkey is low fat, low cholesterol and lower in calories. When you replace turkey for beef or pork in recipes, use fresh herbs such as basil, cilantro, chilies, ginger, tarragon, etc. and bake, broil or grill. Add to sauces, sauté without adding oil. Chicken is lower in fat and calories than other meats, but turkey is even lower.

Turkey can be used in recipes to make dishes like meatloaf, stuffed cabbage, stuffed peppers, pasta dishes, meat sauce, chilies, chow mein, sandwiches and salads.

LOWER FAT COOKING (turkey breast)

Turkey breast - without skin 3 ounces contains about 1 gram of fat, 3 ounces of chicken breast contains about 3 grams of fat.

Turkey cutlets – slices of turkey breast ¼ inch thick; weigh about 2 to 3 ounces each. These are also good alternatives for chicken breast, pork tenderloin slices or veal.

Turkey medallions (round) are cut from turkey breast.

Tenderloins, medallions are 1 inch thick, weigh about 2 to 3 ounces each.

Turkey medallions can be used to substitute pork or veal medallions in recipes.

Turkey steaks – cut from the turkey breast

½ to 1 inch thick

Turkey steak may be baked, broiled, grilled, cut into strips for stir-fry. Cut into pieces for kabobs and ground for turkey burger. Great for chicken recipes.

Ground turkey – Ground turkey can be used in any dish as a substitute for ground beef, chicken, veal or pork.

CHANGE THE RECIPES WHENEVER POSSIBLE TO CUT THE FAT, SAVE ON CALORIES AND ENJOY COMPLEX CARBOHYDRATES

POTATOES

Potatoes are not fattening. You can enjoy potatoes, only if you keep it in the healthy range. Potatoes are high in complex carbohydrates and one of the most nutritious foods. It is full of vitamins and minerals. Avoid taking potatoes out of the healthy state by adding regular gravies, butter, and sauces or toppings such as sour cream, cottage cheese, cheeses, and regular bacon bits, etc. Keep them lower in fat. It's not the potato that is fattening, but the toppings or what you mix into it.

MASHED POTATOES – serve plain or flavored. To add flavor mix in the following:

1. Use fresh or dried herbs

2. Smaller amount of shredded cheese, feta or goat

3. Grated cheese

4. Reduced fat sour cream and fresh chives

5. Roasted garlic

6. Caramelized onions

7. Horseradish, grated

8. Stock, chicken, beef or vegetable, 98-99% fat free

9. Sautéed mushrooms

10. Puree vegetables, carrots, celery, and parsnips

11. Sweet potatoes and white potatoes mash together

12. Stir in a few tablespoons of chopped chili

    (in a jar) and equal amount of your favorite salsa

13. Mash with butter flavored granules

14. Mash with skim milk, low fat milk or evaporated skim milk and grated farm cheese, smaller amount

15. Mash with skim milk, low fat milk or evaporated skim milk and butter-flavored granules

16. Mash with bullion cube

17. Mash with spread. (trans-fatty acid free)

BAKED POTATOES WITH TOPPINGS

1. Lower fat/non-fat sour cream and chives

2. Sauteed mushrooms

3. Steamed mixed vegetables, seasoned

4. Reduced fat cheese, melted

5. Chopped fresh cauliflower and broccoli sauteed with little olive oil, seasoned to taste

6. Steamed broccoli and cauliflower with lower fat melted cheese toppings

7. Toss fresh tomatoes, onions, and oregano with a little olive oil

8. Low fat cottage cheese with chopped chives, onions or scallions

9. Small amount of butter-flavored olive oil and small amount of grated parmesan cheese

10. Low fat cottage cheese, chopped green onions, chopped green bell peppers, diced tomatoes, tossed with lemon juice, season to taste

11. Diced cucumbers, diced tomatoes, diced green peppers tossed with vinegar and fresh lime juice

12. Yellow and green peppers, sliced onions, sauteed with a little olive oil

13. Sauteed chopped broccoli, mushrooms, and onions with olive oil

14. Zucchini and corn toppings, sauteed with olive oil

15. Fresh diced zucchini and tomatoes and onions with lime juice

16. Low fat plain yogurt or non-fat yogurt

17. Top with trans-fatty acid free spread

*To sauté, only coat pan with small amount of oil or coat pan with vegetable spray.

PASTA IS NOT FATTENING, IT IS HOW YOU DRESS IT UP

LIGHTEN UP PASTA SALADS

Some tips for cutting the fat from some of the pasta salads that you already use or to adjust some new recipes:

- Use less dressing, half the amount. Use less oil in salads, add oil to cook salad as close to serving time as possible. Cooked pasta soaks up oil.

- Use more fresh vegetables for flavor without fat. You can also grill them for a better taste before adding to the pasta.

- For pasta salad that call for mayonnaise type dressings, use half the amount or use reduced fat mayonnaise and mix with an equal amount of yogurt for flavor.

- Use low fat sauces, salsa and uncooked tomato sauces and reduce oil or no oil in your pasta dish.

- Fresh or dry herbs with less oil or no oil. Be more creative in providing flavor.

- Use small amount of strong flavored cheeses such as feta, goat and gorconzola. Milder cheese requires more to provide flavor to the pasta dish and also adds more calories.

- In place of some oil based recipes, use lemon juice (small amounts) and a small amount of salt and pepper to taste.

- Pasta dishes that call for eggs, use half the amount of sliced or diced eggs or use two cooked egg whites to 1 egg yolk.

- Recipes that require ham, use ½ the amount or use lean or lower fat 97% fat free, or use Canadian bacon (a low fat meat).

- For pasta and fish recipes that call for shrimps or lobster or both, use half the amount, cut in small pieces and mix in well. This will still give that good flavor, but will save on calories. Fish can be grilled with onion, bell pepper, for more flavor and seasoned to taste. All fish are good. Be creative.

KEEPING THAT SAUCE HEALTHY

FOR THICKENING SOUPS, SAUCES, GRAVY

Instead of relying on the traditional fat-laden roux for thickening sauces and soups, try replacing some or all of the roux with:

1. Pureed or shredded potato

2. Pureed, cooked rice

3. Bread crumbs

4. Cooked cereal mix (rice or wheat)

5. Pureed, cooked beans

6. Pureed vegetables

7. A lighter mixture of cornstarch, arrowroot or flour with de-fated stock

8. Plain flour and water mixture

BREADED VEGETABLES AS A MAIN DISH OR SIDE DISH

Some vegetables can be used to replace meat in recipes like meat chili for vegetable chili. Americans are becoming increasingly aware of the importance of vegetables to their health. Vegetables can be used as a major part of a meal. Vegetables provide a variety of choices, which help a healthy meal plan from getting boring. Rotating vegetables with meat meal will help you lose and maintain your weight.

Example 1:   Breaded vegetables, shake and baked served with baked potato, Homemade reduced fat sour cream, low-fat tomato salsa.

Example 2:   Health salad – breaded vegetables, shake and baked served with veggie burger on a bun or seeded roll, lettuce leaf, cucumber and tomato with mustard.

As the emphasis on providing lower fat items continues to grow and frying foods is now being avoided, breaded vegetables are being used more as a main dish.

Breaded vegetables include: broccoli, cauliflower, green tomatoes, tomatoes, carrots, mushrooms, eggplant, zucchini, yellow squash, butternut and more. Some vegetables may be best to slightly steam first, then bread and bake or grill.

Breaded eggplant parmesan baked with tomato sauce and reduced fat cheese is another good alternative on meatless days. Fresh eggplant breaded with home-made bread crumbs layered with low-fat ricotta cheese and low-fat mozzarella, home-made tomato sauce, salt and pepper with tomato sauce which is a good alternative for veal parmesan.

Other dishes which can be served, as a meal dish is breaded broccoli and/or cauliflower. Just before serving, top with a healthy homemade sauce.

154

Rice and beans can be served with a side dish of half tomato, topped with seasoned bread crumbs with basil, oregano and other fresh herbs and then baked.

Breaded baked vegetables balls of equal parts boiled and mashed, carrots, peas, and potatoes and served in a tomato sauce or other home-made vegetable sauce, three or four balls as a side or main dish. Be creative.

COMBINATION FOODS – HEALTHY COOKING

- Casseroles, use less meat and more vegetables.

- Cheese pizza, use thinner crust, reduces fat or smaller amounts of regular shredded cheese with lots of healthy vegetables.

- Chili with beans – De-fat the ground beef, use the leanest or use lean ground turkey. Use more beans or mixed vegetables and less ground meat. Try also vegetable chili at times.

- Chow mein, stir fry with less oil. Use less meat ½ to 1 oz. per serving.

- Macaroni and cheese – use skim or 1% milk or reduced fat canned milk and reduced fat cheese or half the amount of regular cheese.

- Soup – make vegetable soups without meat or smaller portions of meat. De-fat broth before adding thickening. Make cream soup with 1% milk or skim canned milk.

- Spaghetti and meat sauce – use lean ground meat, drain and watch off excess fat or use lean ground turkey. You may try using less ground meat in the sauce.

- Puddings – Use fat-free or 1% milk only top with fresh fruit (bananas, melon, berries, strawberries, etc.) Makes a nice dessert.

THE FOLLOWING COOKING METHODS ALSO REDUCE CALORIES:

Broiling –   This allows fat to drip from meats, poultry and fish during cooking

Grilling –   Also allows fat to drip from meat, poultry and fish during cooking. If you broil, grill, or barbecue, protect foods from contact with smoke, flame, and extremely high temperatures. Move racks or grills away from heat sources. Cook more slowly, and wrap food in foil or put it in pan before grilling or barbecuing.

Poaching –   Cooking is a low-calorie liquid. It let's you quickly simmer poultry, fish or eggs.

Sautéing -   Let's you cook foods with very little oil.

Spraying Pan with non-stick cooking oil – Coating the pan and sautéing meats and vegetables without adding additional fats. This technique is good for cooking mix dishes when small amount of cooking is needed.

Simmering in water – Instead of sautéing vegetables in fats or oils, per cook vegetables by simmering them in a small amount of water or until vegetables are tender, then drain off excess water and add vegetables to recipes.

The variety of cooking techniques will assist you in maintaining healthy eating habits without counting calories. Many of these cooking methods are also quick so you will not have to spend a lot of time in the kitchen. Many believe that lower fat cooking is time consuming, but this is not necessarily so.

GRILLING KEBABS – Metal skewers are better for grilling kebabs. This type will allow cooking the excess fat to drain off. Alternate marinated meat cubes with your favorite vegetables or fruit or a combination of both.

If you use wood skewers to keep the wood from scorching, wrap both ends of the threaded kebabs with s small piece of heavy-duty foil. Remove foil before serving.

SIMMERING In water and spraying pan with non-stick cooking oil – First spray the pan then add a small amount of water. Add vegetables or sliced or diced potatoes. Cover pan and let vegetables steam. As water reduces out, the vegetables will become tender and begin to brown. This method is good for making home fried potatoes. Reduce heat; let potatoes slightly brown on one side, then turn and brown on the other side.

COATING THE PAN – Take a paper towel and soak with vegetable oil, rub around inside of the pan. You can stir-fry vegetables and or diced meats, poultry or fish. You can also pan fry thin slices of meat, poultry, fish, and vegetables seasoned or slightly floured. This cooking method is good for people who like the taste of fried foods.

DEFATING GROUND BEEF – After sautéing, drain off excess fat from brown ground meat. Use a wire mesh strainer or a metal colander. If you like, you may also wash additional fat away by holding colander or strainer with ground meat under running water.

BARBECUING – This will add flavor to lean cuts of meats, poultry, fish and vegetables such as bell pepper, onions, and eggplants. Direct dry heat will seal in the flavor, juices and provide crispy products.

WRAPPED AND COOKED – Wrap poultry, fish, corn, etc. in foil, parchment paper parcel or place in a sealed roasting bag with chopped vegetables, garlic, herbs, spices, citrus juice or wine. This will provide flavor and moisture. Place in a pan and put in the oven and bake until tender. This method of cooking provides the greatest amount of flavor and moisture.

LOW FAT FRYING – Start by bringing a small amount of water, broth (99% fat free), and wine, liquid from steamed vegetables, or fish, use a non-stick skillet and bring the liquid to a boil. Add the chopped vegetables, meat, poultry, or fish and cook until tender. This will depend on the portion size. Skim off fat if any, and reduce the heat to low. Add a little more liquid if needed. When the item becomes tender, let the water cook out. Turn down the flame and let the item brown on both sides. Some meat, poultry and fish, vegetables can be dry – fried without the added fat in a non-stick skillet over low heat until the food becomes slightly browned.

STEAM – BASKET – Place vegetables, poultry or fish in a steamer basket and set it over a pan of boiling liquid. The liquid can be flavored with garlic or your favorite herbs. Steam until tender and done.

PRE-BOILING TO ADD FLAVOR – Vegetables that need to be pre-cooked before adding to soup, casseroles, or oven-baked dish can be broiled slightly first with garlic or your favorite herbs. Then add to the dish to complete cooking. This will increase the flavor.

MICROWAVE FOR LOW-FAT COOKING – Let's you cook food without adding fat. Try cooking beef in the microwave. Cooking beef in the microwave will allow more fat to drain or drip off. It may take a little practice to get it right.

Tenderloin steaks, top sirloin steaks, flank steaks, top round steaks, tip roasts, eye of the round, and ground beef are suitable for microwave cookery.

Cooking roast or steak – The best setting for most cuts of beef will require a medium-low or medium setting. Collect meat drippings in microwave-safe utensils. Use a rack for roasts and meat loaves. Measure the internal temperature of roasts with a microwave-safe thermometer. If the roast needs to cook a little longer, cook in 30-second increments until the desired doneness is reached.

170°F well done   150°F medium-rare

160°F medium   140°F rare

Setting for cooking ground beef – high.

To brown ground beef, place beef in a colander over a container to catch the drippings.

RECIPES, FOOD PREPARATION AND WEIGHT CONTROL

The ABCD - Eases's of weight loss and maintenance began with food preparation. It is what you add to the food during preparation that adds up to a high fat, high calorie meal. Before planning a menu, chose foods that are lower in fats, foods that provide a good source of protein, complex carbohydrates and foods that are higher in vitamins and minerals. You must be conscious and be more aware of the nutrition content of foods, so it is necessary to read labels for ingredients and nutrient content for fats, sugar and sodium. It is okay to prepare your favorite meal with higher fats or sugary meal once or twice a week to satisfy your needs, then return back to that healthier meal preparation.

Research new healthy recipes, cutting back does not mean cutting out all together. When you do treat yourself to a higher fat or sugary meal, you may need to only eat a smaller portion to satisfy that need. Remember not to let yourself get too hungry before eating for this may cause overeating. Remember eating smaller meals throughout the day is better instead of the three meals a day pattern. Have your salad, broth, or glass of skim milk or tall glass of ice water before you eat.

Before you plan a meal or recipe, make your shopping list and try to avoid buying food items that are high in fat or sugar. You must have as many healthier foods in the house at all times. This will make things easier for you. A meal plan too low in calories is not good for a long period of time. Remember the reverse will occur. You will grow fatter.

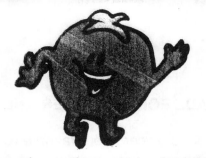

HAVE FUN WITH YOUR RECIPES

Keeping track of your fat grams and counting calories just do not work. The total amount of healthier food you eat for the day or week is better than counting calories or fat grams. Shopping healthier is a must. That is why it is so important to eat a variety of foods. Do your research, try new recipes and learn to change them into lower fat. Make a shopping list. Have a new relationship with foods. Buy a variety of foods. Foods that are lower in total fat, saturated fat and cholesterol. Eat more vegetables, fruits and grain products. Use sugar in moderation. Use salt and sodium products in moderation. The key to healthier recipes and healthy eating is to make sure that you do not over season the foods with higher calorie, high fat or sugary ingredients. If you do not want to use low fat ingredients in some recipes, it may be possible to just try cutting back on the fatty ingredients or de-fat the item before completing the dish.

Remember you do not need will power to eat healthy, lose weight or to keep the weight off. You will only be setting yourself up for failure. When it comes to healthy eating and weight control, all you need is knowledge. Learn how to cook healthy and you will eat healthy without counting calories or fat grams.

If you shop right, you will cook right and you will eat right. It is just that easy. To start with, I am not too concerned about the amount of food you consume, but the type of food you eat and how you prepare it. Lower fat, reduced sugar in cooking is a necessary link for healthy eating, weight loss and maintenance. You may eat the same amount of food and still lose weight. If you start out by eating healthier, in time you will start to cut your food intake too.

TRICKS TO THE TRADE FOR HEALTHIER AND TASTY RECIPES

There is no need to discard your favorite recipe because it may be loaded with fat or sugar. Follow the simple guidelines to help you develop healthy recipes for almost any meal plan.

1. May cook chicken with skin on. Chicken cooked with skin will not absorb the fat from the skin. Cooking with the skin on will retain the moisture and the flavor. Remove the skin before serving will reduce total calories.

2. Remove all visible fat before cooking steak or all other meat, but if meat is lean you can remove fat after cooking.

3. De-fat stock or sauce before completing the dish.

4. Pesto Sauce cut back on the oil and add de-fated broth.

5. Alfredo Sauce – use non-fat ricotta cheese whisked with skim or 1% milk and reduced fat cream cheese and trans fatty acid free butter.

6. Cooked vegetables - add whipped butter or butter substitute just before serving or spray with flavored oil to coat the vegetables.

7. Use skim milk, 1% milk, canned low fat milk or de-fatted broth for mashed potatoes.

8. Avoid using roux to thicken sauce, gravy and soup. Instead add pureed vegetables, mashed potatoes, pureed rice or cornstarch or flour to thicken stocks, etc.

9. To add flavor to grilled foods, add nutshell, herb branches, seeds, fennel stalks, or citrus peels to the coals or wood chips.

10. To lean ground beef add bread, vegetables or fruit as a filler.

11. Use powders or concentrated from or dehydrated foods to add flavor, like beans, fruits, mushrooms, garlic, vegetables, powder.

12. Caramelized onion provide flavor and cut the fat.

13. Make concentrated tea and mix with vinegar in place of oil to season sauce, rice, and seafood or for salad dressings.

14. Lemon preserved or lemon peel provide flavor.

15. Chopped nuts as flavor but add less.

16. Sun-dried fruits added to salad reduced the amount of oil add flavor.

17. Add only small amount of butter to the dishes like soups or potatoes just before serving to trick the taste buds.

18. Steam vegetables with string-flavored herbs.

19. Squeeze fresh lemons or lime over vegetables or soup just before eating for a great taste.

20. Balsamic with less oil provide excellent flavor to salads and vegetables.

CHANGING YOUR RECIPE

To reduce the fat content you can turn a high fat spread into a low fat, low cholesterol feast.

Example – spaghetti and meatballs

A spaghetti meal fat content can be increased from 4 percent to 36 percent just by adding as little as four meatballs per serving. By replacing the ground beef with ground turkey can reduce the fat content by 32 percent per meatball.

Replacement for oil and eggs: When baking, substitute plain non-fat yogurt in place of the oil and eggs. You will get the same moist and good flavor without the added fat and cholesterol and 1/3 less calories.

REPLACING WHOLE EGGS IN RECIPES

1 large egg = 3 tablespoons egg substitute

1 large egg = 1 ½ large egg white

1 large egg = 2 tablespoons egg substitute

BUTTER AND OTHER FAT REPLACEMENT TIPS

1. In place of butter, use a clarified form of butter called ghee.

    Milk solids have been removed to form clarified butter. It is tasty and can be purchased at many health food stores.

2. Make your own homemade clarified butter. (Homemade ghee).

3. Olive oil is also a delicious and healthy butter replacement (Do not over use).

    Olive oil also comes in a spray can, used to stir-fry or sauté, or spray on vegetable, rice, potatoes, pastas, and on toast without adding calories but will add a good flavor.

4. Butter flavored granules will provide a delicious flavor to vegetables, potatoes, rice, pastas, and fish without adding calories.

5. Butter substitute spray can be used for toppings, cooking and basting and will provide zero calories per 1 gram serving.

6. If regular butter, margarine, mayonnaise, salad dressing etc. is used, follow these rules:

    a. instead of 1 tablespoon, use 1 teaspoon

b.   reduce vegetable oil in recipes by one third

7.   For margarine or butter, use non-fat or reduced fat or tran-fatty acid free buttery spreads.

8.   Mayonnaise, use non-fat or reduced fat or smaller amounts of regular mayonnaise or make home-make lower-fat mayonnaise.

9.   For regular salad dressings, use fat-free or reduced fat, which come in many flavors.

CHANGING YOUR RECIPES

VEGETABLE OILS (FOR COOKING AND SEASONING)

It is fine to use some oil in cooking. The amount of oil you choose to cook with at any given time should depend on the level of fat intake for that day or week. Example: If you have had too many high fatty meals for the week, you may want to balance it with lower fat cooking techniques before the end of the week. You can use a little less oil or use an oil spray or combine oil with a little water, fruit juice or broth which is called wet frying and dry frying techniques.

-     Use less oil in vinaigrette   and add a small amount of honey. This will complement the acidity of the vinegar.

-     Vinaigrettes use reduced wine in place of vinegar for flavorful wine friendly salads. The acidity will be lower so you can use less oil in recipes.

-     Use lemongrass because it will replace the flavor that fat provides.

-     Get a spray bottle and fill it with olive oil. One firm spray will coat a pan with a thin even film of oil which can be used for baking, sautéing or stir-fry. This can also be used to spray meat, fish or vegetables before grilling. You can spray slightly hot cooked vegetable just before serving to give that liked texture and flavor. Buy your favorite olive oil; you can also buy buttered flavor vegetable oil.

CHANGING YOUR RECIPES

BAKING WITH OIL IS HEALTHIER

There is no need to discard your favorite recipes that maybe loaded with saturated fat. You can change just about any recipe. Many times you can replace vegetable oil for butter, margarine, shortening or lard in recipes.

FOLLOW THIS OIL CONVERSION CHART:

In place of butter, margarine, shortening, lard	Use Vegetable Oil
1 teaspoon	¾ teaspoon
1 tablespoon	2 ¼ teaspoons
2 tablespoons	1 ½ tablespoons
¼ cup	3 tablespoons
1/3 cup	¼ cup
½ cup	¼ cup + 2 tablespoons
2/3 cup	½ cup
¾ cup	½ cup + 1 tablespoon
1 cup	¾ cup

OTHER TIPS FOR CHANGING RECIPES AND DEFATTING RECIPES

TO CONTROL TOTAL CALORIES:

Choose a cooking method that adds little or no fats to your foods:

Bake, steam, poach, roast, or use a microwave oven.

Choose foods that require little fat. Stir-fry in small amounts of unsaturated vegetable oil.

- When using fat or oil to sauté or stir-fry, use with vegetable oils instead of animal fats, butter, lard, bacon grease.

- Remove fat with an oil separating measuring cup before adding the products together.

- Use vegetable oil sprays or lightly coat pan with vegetable oil.

- Use non-stick pans to brown meat.

- Avoid adding larger amount of fat to food during preparation. Try using herbs and spices to enhance flavor. Use more low fat substitutes.

- When making soups, stew, gravies, etc., let cool, place in the refrigerator and chill. After the fat solidifies on the top, spoon the fat off. Then complete.

- Drain off any fatty liquid from meat after cooking or browning, remove drippings after browning meat.

- Use evaporated skimmed milk in dishes in place of light cream.

- Change the recipe, try to use lower fat or fat-free fillings in sandwiches etc. to avoid higher fat spread. If higher fat spreads are used, just use less. Read the labels. Example: regular mayonnaise – a serving is 1 tablespoon which is 100 calories. On a sandwich as a spread to you really need the full serving or would a teaspoon do?

- When a recipe calls for high fat meat, try to choose extra lean cuts of meat and trim off all visible fat and at times, remove skin from poultry. If you enjoy the skin of the chicken at times, enjoy it. The treat will help you stay with a healthy eating plan.

- Recipes that call for whole meat like stewed chicken and rice at times diced the chicken, whole meat required larger portions. So practice balancing your meal. Cut meat up into 1 to 2 ounce portions per serving and add more rice or vegetables, pasta or beans to a mixed dish. Change or modify the recipe for healthier eating.

- In recipes, salad, etc. use white meat of chicken or turkey (white meat contains less fat than dark meat). This does not mean never to eat the dark meat chicken.

- If a recipe calls for stir-fry, use a non-stick Wok or a sauté pan and only a small amount of oil.

- Recipes that call for high sugar content making some changes if possible and cut the sugar.

- For a soup and sandwich meal, change the garnish; serve fresh fruit like orange slices, apple slices, strawberries or grapes as a side dish instead of potato chips or French fries.

- Some fried food dishes like French fry potatoes try changing the recipe to baked French fry potatoes in the oven instead of frying in oil. Use non-stick baking sheet/pan, and spray the pan with vegetable oil.

Other ways to change recipes when cooking potatoes are as follows:

- Drain excess fat from browned or sautéed ground meat before completing recipe.

    - Use low fat and non-fat toppings on baked potato.

    - Mash potatoes with skim milk and whipped butter or tran-fatty acid free

168

- Use Ghee (a clarified form of butter) from a health food store.

- Mash potatoes with homemade clarified butter.

- Add garlic, grated horseradish or butter flavored granules for extra flavor.

- Mash potatoes with olive oil in place of butter.

- Recipes that call for cheese, try reducing the amount.

- Use cheese sprinkle to season vegetables, baked potatoes, salad or pasta. Use any kind of cheese; a sprinkle of cheese will add flavor and only give a small amount of fat, but do not use large amounts of regular cheese for cheese melt sandwiches or toppings.

FOOD SEASONING SUGGESTIONS

To avoid extra fat and calories, try to change the recipes by using no-fat flavorings. These suggested herbs, spices, seasonings and creative cooking provide flavor without adding fat:

BEEF - Nutmeg, onions, onion powder, bay leaf, dry mustard, pepper, all spices, caraway seed, garlic clove or powder, cumin seed, curry powder, ginger, oregano, mushrooms, sage, unsalted canned tomato juice, unsalted puree tomatoes, marjoram, broiled peaches, green pepper, thyme, basil, chili powder.

LAMB - Oregano, lemon juice, garlic, garlic powder, unsalted canned tomato juice, rosemary, thyme, basil, curry, unsalted puree tomatoes, and baked with pineapple ring, dill, mint.

VEAL - Bay leaf, ginger, unsalted canned tomato juice, unsalted puree tomatoes, baked with apricots, marjoram, oregano, rosemary, thyme, garlic, mushrooms, paprika, dill, and sage.

CHICKEN AND TURKEY - Sage, paprika, onion, poultry seasoning, cranberry sauce, cooking with fruits and added flavor (baked with peaches, apples, etc.), rosemary, thyme, basil, mushrooms, bay leaf, coriander, curry garlic, ginger, marjoram, oregano, tarragon.

FISH - Lemon juice, dry mustard, paprika, bay leaves, chives, coriander, dill, nutmeg, sage, tarragon, thyme.

SHELLFISH - Bay leaf, basil, chervil, coriander, curry powder, cloves, dill, marjoram, oregano, tarragon, thyme, onion, lemon, parsley, unsalted canned tomato juice, unsalted puree tomatoes, green pepper, dills.

EGGS - Dry mustard, green pepper, paprika, tomatoes, unsalted puree tomatoes, curry, onions, parsley, thyme, mushrooms, chives, cumin seed, curry powder, savory, tarragon.

PORK - Apples, applesauce, clove, garlic cloves or powder, onions, onion powder, oregano, sage, savory, thyme, caraway seeds, chili, coriander, cumin, curry, dill.

Recipes are only a guide, try other seasonings and be creative.

SEASONING SUGGESTIONS YOU CAN MAKE AHEAD OF TIME

PRE-BLENDED SEASONINGS RESTRICTION:

NOTE: Store away in a dry place away from light.

ITALIAN HERBS:

> 3 tbsp dried oregano
> 3 tbsp dried basil
> 2 tbsp dried marjoram
> 2 tsp dried parsley flakes

PAPRIKA BLEND:

¼ cup paprika
½ tsp dried basil
¼ tsp cayenne
¼ tsp dried marjoram
¼ tsp black pepper
2 tsp salt
(good for casserole, chicken, fish or in salad dressing)

SEASONING SALT:

5 to 6 tbsp salt
½ tsp dried thyme leaves
½ tsp dried marjoram
¼ tsp garlic powder
2 tbsp onion powder
1 tsp curry powder
1 tsp dry mustard
(good for seasoning meats, stews, salads or salad dressing)

SEASONING FOR MEAT AND VEGETABLES:

A.   2 tsp grated lemon peel
1 tsp garlic powder
1 tsp dried thyme
¼ tsp salt
¼ tsp pepper

B.   2 tbs chili powder
2 tsp ground cumin
1 tsp ground oregano
½ tsp ground black pepper
1 tsp garlic powder
1 tsp paprika

SPICY SEASONINGS:

A.   2 tbs garlic powder
2 tbs ground black pepper
2 tbs ground red pepper
2 tbs salt

B.   1 tsp ground oregano
       1 tsp ground rosemary
       1 tsp garlic powder
       1 tsp dry ground basil
       1 tsp salt

MARINADE SAUCE:

ORIENTAL -   1 tsp grated fresh ginger
             ½ tsp ground red pepper
             2 tbs diced onion
             ½ cup lemon juice
             2 tbs vegetable oil
             2 tbs soy sauce

BARBEQUE -   ½ cup catsup
             ½ cup vinegar
             2 tbs sugar
             1 tsp onion powder
             1 tbs vegetable oil
             ½ tsp black pepper
             2 tbs water

             Mix all ingredients together.

REDUCED FAT DIPS FOR THE HEALTHY DIPPER

BASIC HOME-MADE SOUR CREAM MADE WITH YOGURT:

½ cup low-fat yogurt

1 ½ teaspoon lemon juice

Blend until smooth.

BASIC HOME-MADE SOUR CREAM MADE WITH COTTAGE CHEESE:

½ cup low-fat cottage cheese

1 ½ teaspoon lemon juice

Blend until smooth.

EASY HOMEMADE MAYONNAISE:

½ cup low-fat yogurt, or non-fat

½ cup low-fat cottage cheese

1/8 teaspoon salt

Blend until smooth.

MOCK SOUR CREAM:

1 cup low-fat cottage cheese

1 tablespoon skim milk

2 tablespoons lemon juice

Blend until smooth.

YOGURT DIP:

1 cup low-fat plain yogurt or non-fat

¼ cup low-fat mayonnaise

½ teaspoon lemon or lime juice

Blend until smooth.

ITALIAN STYLE YOGURT DIP:

1 cup low-fat plain yogurt or non-fat

¼ cup low-fat mayonnaise

½ teaspoon lemon juice

¼ cup chopped sun dried tomato

½ teaspoon dried oregano

1/8 teaspoon pepper

Blend until smooth.

THOUSAND ISLAND DRESSING (LOW FAT):

1 cup low-fat cottage cheese

1/3 cup ketchup

2 tablespoon chopped onion

1 tablespoon lemon juice

½ cup sweet relish

1. Blend all ingredients except relish.

2. Add sweet relish, mix and chill.

NO FAT SALAD DRESSING:

COMBINE: Dijon Mustard

Chopped Shallots

Fresh herbs

Raspberry vinegar

Lots of fresh lime juice

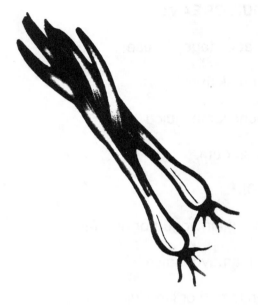

The mustard creates an emulsion that makes the dressing look and taste like it has oil.

TYPE I – HOME-MADE SOUR CREAM:

1 cup low-fat cottage cheese

2 tablespoons lemon juice

Blend together until smooth.

TYPE II – SOUR CREAM DIPS:

1 cup reduced fat sour cream

1 tablespoon skim milk or 1% fat milk

2 tablespoons lemon juice

Blend all ingredients together. Mix and chill.

CORN DIP:

1-12 oz. can whole kernel corn, drained

¼ cup diced onion

1 large tomato chopped

1 jalapeno pepper chopped, no seeds

2 tablespoons low fat mayonnaise

Mix all ingredients together, chill.

DILL SOUR CREAM DIP #1:

1-cup low-fat cottage cheese

1-tablespoon skim milk or 1% milk

2 tablespoons lemon juice

½ teaspoon dill

Blend until smooth.

SPINACH DIP

2 cups plain low-fat yogurt

¼ cup cooked chilled spinach

¼ cup chopped fresh parsley

¼ chopped onion

1/8-teaspoon pepper

Blend until smooth.

FRUIT DIP:

1-cup plain low-fat yogurt or non-fat

¼ cup peach or apricot or strawberry preserve

1/8-teaspoon ground nutmeg

1/8-teaspoon ground cinnamon

Blend until smooth.

DILL SOUR CREAM DIP #2:

½ teaspoon fresh dill diced

1 teaspoon diced onions

1 cup reduced fat sour cream or homemade low fat sour cream

Blend all ingredients together. Mix and chill.

PLAIN YOGURT DIP:

1-cup low-fat plain yogurt or non-fat

¼ cup low-fat mayonnaise

½ teaspoon lemon juice

Blend together and chill.

You may add the following:

1. Sliced or diced fresh fruit (melon, bananas, strawberry, berries, mango, etc.).

2. Add fruit spread, blend in.

3. Add fruit spread, sprinkle with cinnamon or nutmeg or both.

4. Diced dried fruit.

5. A few drops of vanilla flavoring.

CLAM DIP:

1 ½ oz. can mince clam, drained

¼ cup clam juice

8 oz. low-fat cheese cream

1 tablespoon chopped onion

¼ teaspoon salt

6 to 8 drops of Tabasco

1/8 teaspoon of garlic powder

Put all ingredients into blender and blend for 15 seconds. Stop. Stir down with spatula

and blend for another 10 seconds.

GUACAMOLE (AVOCADO IS A GOOD FAT):

1 ripe avocado, pitted and quartered

½ medium onion

1/8-teaspoon garlic powder

1 ripe medium tomato

1-tablespoon olive oil

3 tablespoon lemon juice

1/8-teaspoon salt

1/8-teaspoon pepper

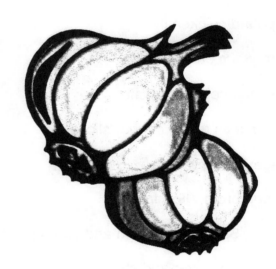

Put all ingredients into the blender and puree for about 30 seconds.

Stop and stir down with spatula and puree for another 30 seconds or until creamy.

WORCESTERSHIRE SAUCE DIP:

1-cup low-fat cottage cheese

1 to 2 tablespoons Worcestershire sauce

¼ cup chopped onions

¼ cup chopped green pepper

¼ teaspoon garlic powder

2 tablespoons lemon juice

1/8-teaspoon ground pepper

Dash of tobasco sauce

Blend until smooth.

CHOPPED CHICKEN LIVER:

In this recipe, butter and oil dripping has been eliminated thus reducing the fat.

1 pound chicken liver

1 medium onion sliced

salt and pepper to taste

½ medium green pepper sliced

vegetable spray

½ cup broth, 99% fat free

- Sauté liver, onion and green pepper with vegetable spray. Cook until tender. Cool liver and chop.

- Place liver mixture into blender, add salt, pepper and 4 tablespoons of fat-free broth. Cover and blend for about 10 seconds.

- Add more broth for a smoother consistency if desired. Blend for another 10 seconds. Do not over blend or puree.

NOTE: High Cholesterol

STRAWBERRIES/CREAM CHEESE TOPPING:

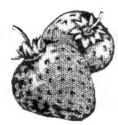

4 oz. low-fat cream cheese, cut up

½ cup evaporated skim milk or low fat

1-pint strawberries (10 oz. frozen) or fresh strawberries

-     Put low-fat cheese and evaporated skim milk into a blender. Blend until smooth.

-     Spoon over strawberries or other fruit and serve.

LOW-FAT GRAVY:

Chill meat dripping and remove all fat with a spoon, then add flour or cornstarch and water as desired for thickness of gravy. Season and simmer.

SHRIMP DIP:

2 cups diced cooked shrimp

½ cup low-fat yogurt

1-cup low-fat cottage cheese

1 ½ teaspoon lemon juice

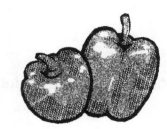

¼ cup finely diced green bell pepper

1 tablespoon prepared horseradish

as needed chicken broth (98-99% fat free)

Salt and pepper to taste.

In blender add: yogurt, cottage cheese and lemon juice together. Blend until smooth.

Add to mixture all other ingredients. Mix and chill.

ONION DIP:

½ cup diced onions

½ cup low-fat yogurt

1-cup low-fat cottage cheese

1 ½ teaspoon lemon juice

1 tablespoon prepared mustard

1 clove garlic, crushed

In blender, add all ingredients until almost smooth, chill.

PESTO DIP:

1 pkg. (10 oz) frozen chopped spinach, thaw well and drain.

½ cup low-fat yogurt

½ cup low-fat cottage cheese

1 ½ teaspoon lemon juice

1/3 cup grated parmesan cheese

¼ cup chopped walnuts

1 clove garlic, crushed

Salt to taste.

In blender, blend all ingredients together, but not too smooth.

BACON DIP:

½ cup diced cooked Canadian bacon

½ cup low-fat yogurt

1-cup low-fat cottage cheese

1 ½ teaspoon lemon juice

¼ cup prepared horseradish

Add yogurt, cottage cheese and lemon juice together in blender. Blend until smooth.

Add in diced bacon and horseradish to mixture. Stir until well mixed.

RECIPE MAKEOVER – TRY IT, YOU MAY LIKE IT

Do not discard your favorite recipes. Try to make changes that will make the recipes have fewer total calories, healthier and still retain its good taste. This book is not loaded with a lot of recipes. It is not a recipe book. However, I did provide a few recipes to show you how to exchange products to save on total calories. These ideas for menu makeovers will allow you to eat your favorite foods without counting calories.

If you do not tell your family and friends about the new healthier recipe changes that is lower in fat, sugar and total calories, they will probably never know. I enjoy trying new recipes makeovers and now I let my family and friends know and they look forward to trying the new recipes knowing that they can enjoy the meal without counting fat grams or calories.

SAUSAGE MACARONI DINNER

REGULAR RECIPE	RECIPE MAKEOVER

1 lb. bulk pork sausage,
   cut into ½" slices
	1 lb. bulk turkey sausage reduced fat
	   cut into ½" slices

1 (16 oz.) can tomatoes, cut up	1 (16 oz.) can tomatoes, cut up
Water	Water
3 tblsp. cooking oil	2 tblsp. vegetable oil
1 cup chopped green pepper	Nonstick cooking spray
1 cup chopped onion	1 cup chopped green pepper
1 (7 ¼ oz.) pkg. macaroni and cheese dinner mix	1 cup chopped onion
¼ cup butter or regular margarine	1 (7 ¼ oz.) pkg. macaroni and cheese dinner mix
½ cup milk	¼ cup tran fatty acid free (smart balance)
	½ cup 1% milk or skim milk

Spray nonstick skillet with cooking spray. Over medium heat, cook sausage until brown on both sides. After sausage is done, remove from skillet and remove fat, if any. Wash out skillet. Drain tomatoes, reserving juice. Add enough water to tomato juice to make 2 ¼ cups. Set aside. Heat oil in same skillet over medium heat. Add green pepper and onion. Sauté 2 minutes. Stir in tomatoes and 2-¼ cup tomato liquid. Cover and cook until mixture comes to a boil, about 1 minute. Stir in macaroni from dinner mix. Reduce heat to low (220°). Cover and simmer 10 minutes, stirring occasionally, until macaroni is tender and liquid is absorbed. Stir in tran fatty acid free, milk and cheese sauce mix from dinner. Add sausage and heat 2 minutes. Makes 4 servings.

CHICKEN WITH RICE (ARROZ CON POLLO)

REGULAR RECIPE	RECIPE MAKEOVER
1 broiler-fryer chicken, (2 to 3 lbs.) cut in pieces	1 broiler-fryer chicken, (2 to 3 lbs.) cut in pieces, remove skin and fat
¼ cup chicken fat	¼ cup vegetable oil
½ cup chopped onion	½ cup chopped onion
1 clove garlic, minced	1 clove garlic, minced
1 large tomato, chopped	1 large tomato, chopped
3 cups hot water	3 cups hot water or chicken broth, 99% fat free
1 cup uncooked rice	1 cup uncooked rice
1 tablespoon minced parsley	1 tablespoon minced parsley
2 teaspoons salt	salt and pepper to taste
½ teaspoon paprika	½ teaspoon paprika
¼ teaspoon pepper	¼ teaspoon saffron
¼ teaspoon saffron	1 bay leaf
1 bay leaf	

Rinse chicken and pat dry with absorbent paper.
Heat oil in a skillet over medium heat. Add onion and garlic;
Cook until onion is tender. Remove with a slotted spoon; set aside.
Put chicken pieces in skillet. Turn to brown pieces on all sides.
When chicken is browned, add tomato, onion, water, rice, parsley, and dry seasonings.
Cover and cook over low heat about 45 minutes, or until thickest pieces of chicken are
tender when pierced with a fork. Remove bay leaf before serving. (Serves 6 to 8).

CONSOMME WITH OXTAILS

REGULAR RECIPE	RECIPE MAKEOVER
3 tablespoons olive oil	*1 medium oxtail (about 4 lbs.) trim off fat
1 medium oxtail (about 4 lbs.)	8 large tomatoes, peeled and seeded
8 large tomatoes, peeled and seeded	2 medium onions
2 medium onions	*2 quart beef broth 99% fat free
2 quarts beef broth	Freshly ground pepper
Freshly ground pepper	Coarse salt
Coarse salt	1 large garlic clove, crushed in a garlic press
1 large garlic clove, crushed in a garlic press	Sprig fresh basil or 1/8 teaspoon dried basil
Sprig fresh basil or 1/8 teaspoon dried basil	1 cup sliced carrot
1 cup sliced carrot	1 cup fresh peas
1 cup fresh peas	4 plantains, boiled
4 plantains, boiled	

*Add oxtail to kettle. Add enough water to cover oxtail. Add a little salt to water. Cook for about 1-½ hours over medium heat. Remove oxtail from liquid with a slotted spoon; set aside. Discard liquid and wash all fat from kettle. Put oxtails back in kettle, add broth. Mince tomatoes, onions and seasonings. Add carrot and peas; continue to cook until meat easily comes from the bones. Add plantain in half to pot. Let cook until firm and tender. Serve consommé with a piece of meat and a plantain half in each soup plate. (Serves 8).

COLD ASPARAGUS SOUP

REGULAR RECIPE	RECIPE MAKEOVER
¾ lb. asparagus, cut up or 1 10-ounce pkg. frozen cut asparagus	¾ lb. asparagus, cut up or 1 10-ounce pkg. frozen cut asparagus
1 thin slice onion	1 thin slice onion
½ cup boiling water	½ cup boiling water
1 cup milk	*1 cup milk 1% or skim
½ cup light cream	½ cup canned milk low fat or skim milk

In covered saucepan cook asparagus and onion slice in water 8 to 10 minutes or till crisp-tender; do not drain. Cool slightly. In blender container or food processor combine the un-drained asparagus and onion, milk, cream, ½ teaspoon salt, and dash pepper. Cover and blend till smooth. Chill for 3 to 4 hours. Stir or blend before serving. (Serves 4 to 6).

POTATO-TOMATO SOUP

REGULAR RECIPE	RECIPE MAKEOVER
4 cups cubed potatoes	4 cups cubed potatoes
3 medium tomatoes, peeled and chopped (2 cups)	3 medium tomatoes, peeled and chopped (2 cups)
1 cup chopped carrot	1 cup chopped carrot
1 cup chopped celery	1 cup chopped celery
3 10 ½ ounces cans condensed beef broth	3 10 ½ ounces cans beef broth 99% fat free
1 small bay leaf	1 small bay leaf
2 slices pumpernickel bread	2 slices pumpernickel bread
1 cup dairy sour cream	1 cup sour cream, reduced fat or fat free
Salt and pepper to taste	Salt and pepper to taste

In large saucepan combine first 6 ingredients. Bring to boil. Reduce heat; cover and simmer 20 minutes or till vegetables are tender.

Meanwhile, cube bread; place bread cubes on baking sheet. Toast in 350° oven 10 minutes; set aside. Remove bay leaf from soup. Top each serving with toast cubes and a dollop of sour cream. Makes 8 servings.

BEEF WITH EGGPLANT

REGULAR RECIPE	RECIPE MAKEOVER
1 lb. ground chuck	¾ lb. ground chuck, lean
½ cup chopped onion	½ cup chopped onion
¼ cup chopped green pepper	¼ cup chopped green pepper
1 clove garlic, minced	1 clove garlic, minced
1 tblsp. flour	1 tblsp. flour
1 (8 oz.) can tomato sauce	1 (8 oz.) can tomato sauce
¾ cup water	¾ cup water
½ tsp. salt	salt and pepper to taste
½ tsp. dried oregano leaves	½ tsp. dried oregano leaves
½ tsp. chili powder	½ tsp. chili powder
1/8 tsp. pepper	1 small unpared eggplant,
1 small unpared eggplant,	cut into ½" slices (1 lb.)
cut into ½" slices (1 lb.)	¾ cup shredded Cheddar cheese
1 cup shredded Cheddar cheese	reduced fat or part skim milk
2 tblsp. chopped fresh parsley	2 tblsp. chopped fresh parsley

Measure all ingredients before starting to cook. Cook ground chuck, onion, green pepper and garlic in 12" skillet over medium heat until browned, discard fat, if any. Stir in flour, tomato sauce, water, salt, oregano, chili powder and pepper. Arrange eggplant slices on top. Reduce heat to low (220°). Cover and simmer 7 minutes or until eggplant is tender. Sprinkle with cheese. Cover and cook 2 minutes or until cheese is melted. Sprinkle with parsley before serving. Makes 4 servings.

CHILI con CARNE

REGULAR RECIPE	RECIPE MAKEOVER
1 ½ lbs. ground beef	1 lb. lean ground beef or less
1 large onion, chopped	1 large onion, chopped
1 clove garlic, minced	1 clove garlic, minced
4 cups (two 16 oz. cans) cooked tomatoes	4 cups (two 16 oz. cans) cooked tomatoes
2 cups (one 15 oz. can) red kidney beans	3 cups (one 15 oz. can) red kidney beans
1 tablespoon chili powder	1 tablespoon chili powder
salt and pepper to taste	salt and pepper to taste
¼ teaspoon pepper	¼ teaspoon pepper

Cook ground beef in a large skillet, stirring until crumbled into small pieces and well browned. Remove fat, if any. Add onion and garlic to meat; cook about 5 minutes, stirring frequently. Add tomatoes to skillet and chop into bite-size chunks. Stir in kidney beans, chili powder, salt, and pepper. Reduce heat to simmering and cook, stirring occasionally, about 30 minutes. Serves 6 to 8.

HAM AND PEA SOUP

REGULAR RECIPE	RECIPE MAKEOVER

2 11¼ oz. cans condensed green
   pea soup
1 cup chicken broth
2 cups milk
1 6¾ oz. can chunk-style ham, drained
and diced, or 1 cup diced fully cooked ham
1 2 oz. can mushroom stems and pieces
¼ cup dry white wine
	*2 11¼ oz. cans condensed green
	   pea soup reduced fat, 99% fat free, low
	   salt, low fat
	*1 cup chicken broth 98-99% fat free
	*2 cups 1% milk or skim canned milk
	*1 cup Canadian bacon or lean canned
	   cured or boiled ham, diced fully cooked
	1 2 oz can mushroom stems and pieces
	¼ cup dry white wine

In saucepan combine pea soup and chicken broth; stir in milk. Cook and stir till heated through. Stir in ham, un-drained mushrooms, and wine; heat through. Serves 4 to 6.

TACOS

REGULAR RECIPE	RECIPE MAKEOVER
1/3 cup chopped onion 1 clove garlic, minced 1 lb. ground chuck beef 2 tblsp. chili powder 1 tsp. salt ½ tsp. ground cumin 1 tsp. sugar 2 drops Tabasco sauce 1 cup water 2 tblsp. taco sauce 12 taco shells 1 cup shredded Cheddar cheese 1 cup shredded lettuce 1 large tomato, chopped	1/3 cup chopped onion 1 clove garlic, minced *1 lb. ground chuck, lean or turkey breast 2 tblsp. chili powder salt and pepper to taste ½ tsp. ground cumin 1 tsp. sugar 2 drops Tabasco sauce 1 cup water 2 tblsp. taco sauce 12 taco shells *1 cup shredded Cheddar cheese reduced fat or 2% milk 1 cup shredded lettuce 1 large tomato, chopped

Cook ground chuck, onion and garlic in 10" skillet over medium-high heat 8 minutes or until browned. Drain off excess fat, if any.

Meanwhile, cut and measure remaining ingredients. Add chili powder, salt, cumin, sugar, Tabasco sauce, water and taco sauce to skillet. Cook until mixture comes to a boil, about 1 minute.

Reduce heat to low. Simmer, uncovered, 15 minutes or just until liquid is reduced.

Spoon some of meat mixture into each taco shell. Top each with cheese, lettuce and tomato. Makes 12 tacos or 6 servings.

LOW-CAL VEGETABLE OMELET

REGULAR RECIPE	RECIPE MAKEOVER
1 cup peeled carrot strips, 2" lengths ½ cup sliced onion 3 tblsp. butter or regular margarine 1 cup sliced fresh mushrooms 8 eggs ¼ cup milk salt and pepper to taste 2 tblsp. butter or regular margarine	1 cup peeled carrot strips, 2" lengths ½ cup sliced onion 2 tblsp. vegetable oil or trans fatty acid free smart balance 1 cup sliced fresh mushrooms *4 whole eggs *4 egg whites *¼ cup 1% milk or skim milk or low fat ev. 2 tblsp. vegetable oil or trans fatty acid free salt and pepper to taste

Dice and measure carrots and onion. Slice mushrooms, 2 tblsp. oil in 10" skillet over medium heat. Add carrots, onion, mushrooms and salt to skillet and saute until tender. Combine eggs, milk, salt and pepper in bowl, beat until blended.

Remove vegetables to another bowl from skillet. 2 tblsp. oil in same skillet over low heat. Pour eggs into skillet. As egg mixture sets, lift with spatula to allow uncooked portions to flow to bottom of skillet. Cook until egg is completely set. Loosen edges of omelet. Spoon cooked vegetables over omelet. Fold in half and remove to serving platter. Makes 4 servings.

NOTE: Some trans fatty and acid free may not melt well so I recommend smart balance.

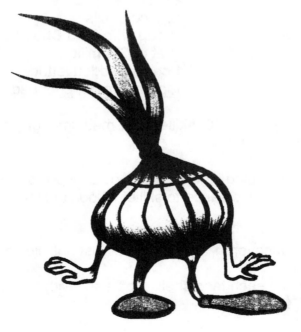

SALAD AS A PRE-MEAL OR SNACK

TOPPING FOR COOKED VEGETABLE (NOT ONLY FOR SALAD)

Vegetable can be seasoned to taste or cooked and topped with Smart Balance buttery spread or sprinkled with some many fat-free, reduced fat salad dressings. (Do your homework). *Fat-free Italian, Zesty Italian, Thousand Island, French and many more.

*Vegetable toppings – Balsamic vinegar, white vinegar, cider vinegar, ketchup, lemon juice, lime juice, herds sauted crushed garlic, sauted onion, Dijon mustard and many more sauces and dressings.

HOMEMADE VEGETABLE TOPPINGS

SHALLOTS – VINAIGRETTE

1 tablespoons olive oil
¼ cup wine vinegar
1 tablespoons chopped parsley
1 tablespoons finely chopped shallots
salt and pepper to taste
Combine all ingredients together.

RECOMMENDED FOR:

-   Kale

-   Raw spinach

-   Swiss chard

-   Toss salad

-   Kidney beans

-   Black beans

MINT-VINAIGRETTE DRESSING

2 tablespoons olive oil
¼ cup wine vinegar
1 tablespoon fresh mint, finely chopped
salt and pepper to taste
Combine all the ingredients together.

RECOMMENDED FOR:

- Carrots cooked, raw or carrot salad

- Sweet onion

- Brussel sprouts

- Cabbage

- Tofu

CURRY VINAIGRETTE DRESSING

1 tablespoon olive oil
¼ cup wine vinegar
2 tablespoon lemon juice
2 teaspoon Dijon mustard
2 teaspoons curry powder
2 teaspoons Splenda
garlic powder
salt and pepper
Combine all the ingredients together.

RECOMMENDED FOR:

- Asparagus

- Kale

- Raw spinach

- Kidney beans

- Black beans

- Swiss chard

- Millet and beans

PAPRIKA VINAIGRETTE DRESSING

¼ cup wine vinegar
1 tablespoon olive oil
2 teaspoons Dijon mustard
1 teaspoon Splenda
¼ teaspoon paprika
garlic powder
Combine all the ingredients together.

RECOMMENDED FOR:

- Green beans

- Wax beans

- Spinach

- Kale

- Cabbage

- Potatoes

- Green beans and almonds

MUSTARD – BROWN RICE VINAIGRETTE DRESSING

¼ cup brown rice vinegar
1 teaspoon olive oil
1 teaspoon Splenda
1 tablespoon Dijon mustard
Combine all ingredients together.

RECOMMENDED FOR:

- Brussels sprouts

- Cabbage

- Carrots

- Tofu

FRENCH VINAIGRETTE DRESSING

1 tablespoon olive oil
2 tablespoon wine vinegar
1 tablespoon lemon juice
½ teaspoon Splenda
garlic powder
salt and pepper
Combine all the ingredients together.

RECOMMENDED FOR:

- Spinach, broccoli

- Green beans

- Marinated vegetables

- Salads

- Pasta salad

- Tomatoes

- Beans

BALSAMIC VINAIGRETTE DRESSING

¼ cup balsamic vinegar
1 tablespoon olive oil
½ teaspoon Splenda
garlic powder
salt and pepper
Combine all the ingredients together.

RECOMMENDED FOR:

- Steamed vegetables

- Vegetables salad

- Green salad

- Pasta salad

SESAME – BROWN RICE DRESSING

¼ cup brown rice vinegar
¼ cup dark sesame oil
2 teaspoons low sodium soy sauce
1 teaspoon Splenda
salt and pepper
Combine all the ingredients together.

RECOMMENDED FOR:

- Brown rice

- Brussels Sprouts

- Cabbage

- Green beans

- Mixed vegetables

HERB VINAIGRETTE DRESSING

¼ cup olive oil
2 tablespoons wine vinegar
1 tablespoon lemon juice
2 teaspoons Dijon mustard
1 teaspoon Splenda
onion powder
dried parsley flakes
dried oregano
dried thyme
salt and pepper
Combine all the ingredients together.

RECOMMENDED FOR:

- Green salad

- Vegetable salad

- Hot potato salad

- Cold potato salad

CIDER VINAIGRETTE DRESSING

1 tablespoon olive oil
¼ cup apple cider vinegar
1 tablespoon Splenda
¼ teaspoon dry mustard
onion powder
paprika
salt
Combine all the ingredients together.

RECOMMENDED FOR:

- Steamed broccoli, cauliflower, spinach

- Green salad

- Mushrooms

- Barley

CHILI LIME DRESSING

2 tablespoons olive oil
2 tablespoon lime juice
1 teaspoon chili powder
½ teaspoon Splenda
garlic powder
Combine all the ingredients together.

RECOMMENDED FOR:

- Corn

- Succatash

- Lima beans

- Broccoli

- Beans

PLUM VINAIGRETTE DRESSING

¼ cup plum vinegar
1 tablespoon olive oil
salt and pepper
Combine all the ingredients together.

RECOMMENDED FOR:

-   Kale

-   Spinach

-   Dandelion greens

-   Collard greens

-   Green peas

-   Onions

-   Green salad

SECTION E – PART I

WHY EXERCISE OR INCREASE PHYSICAL ACTIVITIES?

SECTION-E COMPLIMENTS A HEALTHY EATING REGIMEN

A light exercise program is a must during weight loss and maintenance. This will help you lose weight, burn fat, calories and tone the body. Exercise or increased physical activity will also help you maintain your weight within a normal range. As we age, it will help us maintain a good muscle tone. It will improve your digestive system and improve your mental state, stabilize your blood sugar and you will also look and feel your best.

Sections A, B, C, D, and E, makes it A, B, C, D, Easy to eat healthier for life and maintain a more healthier weight for you. You shouldn't do one without the other. Eating healthier and exercising or increased physical activities both will help raise your metabolic rate.

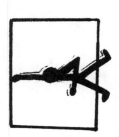

SETPOINT

It is believed that there is a setting inside our body that regulates our weight. This setting is called the "set point." The body defends this "set point". If you persist with a low calorie diet, the body lowers its metabolic rate so that you burn fewer calories. You will stop losing weight unless you change your set point. You can begin to start losing weight by changing or resetting your set point by exercising. You do not need an enormous amount of exercise. Moderate exercise will burn up calories and speed up the rate at which calories are burned.

- Bicycling
- Walking (brisk)
- Dancing
- Jogging
- Jumping
- Jumping rope
- Swimming

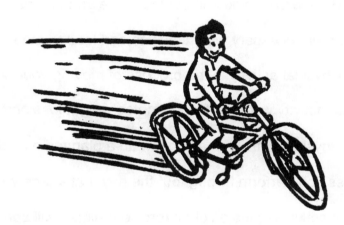

Healthy meal plan, exercise, activity, and behavior modifications are still the mainstay of long-term weight control. Some researchers are studying drugs that appear to burn fat, regardless of what is eaten or how much. These studies are still in their early stages but there are many herbs that help burn off fat and appear to replace it with muscle tissue.

PHYSICAL ACTIVITY PROMOTES HEALTH

Physical activity promotes loss of fat and development of muscles. You gain weight because of lack of physical activity. You need to start moving again. Your sedentary life style is causing the body metabolism to slow down and you burn less fat and you will start to gain weight, as you get older. The amount of muscle in your body tend to decline. The percentage of fat may increase with age and metabolism may decrease with age. So you may need to eat less and become more active throughout life.

By age 35, if you still eat the same and decrease your physical activities, you may gain unnecessary weight, which can lead to other health problems.

Physical activity is the process of moving your body and using your muscles. Physical activity will burn fat, promotes weight loss and maintenance.

• Physical activity does not mean a planned exercise regimen, but it is the various activities you perform throughout the day that keeps your body moving. Increased daily physical activities plus a light exercise regimen will speed up your metabolic and burn calories and this will change your set point.

EXERCISE REGIMEN IS NECESSARY.

Select a light exercise program or sport or increase physical activity.

EXAMPLE: For the beginner, out of shape, or extremely overweight, do the following:

• ☐ Light walking

• ☐ Fun dancing

• ☐ Light stationary bike

- ☐ Treadmill

- ☐ If you are extremely overweight or have been inactive for any long period of time, you may want to start out by following the light stationary, toning exercises.

For more advanced workout, do the following:

- ☐ Brisk walking

- ☐ Bicycling

- ☐ Jogging

- ☐ Jumping rope

- ☐ Swimming

- ☐ Add strength training for muscle mass (muscle burns fat)

NOTE: Consult your physician, especially if you were inactive any length of time.

He/she will determine whether or not you have any illness, which may restrict you from some type of exercise.

Write down the types of exercise/activity that you will enjoy. It doesn't have to be any of the listed above.

_____

_____

_____

_____

_____

_____

_____

PHYSICAL ACTIVITY THAT WILL HELP YOU KEEP MOVING:

1.   Get off the bus a few stops before and walk the rest of the way.

2.   Ride a bike to the store, leave the car parked.

3.   Park the car further away in the parking lot when shopping.

4.   Clean your house yourself, wash windows, vacuum and mop.

5.   Walk up the stairs throughout the day as many times as you can.

6.   Plant in the garden and weed it yourself.

7.   Have fun cooking your own healthy meal. Move back and forward to get the
        ingredients.

8.   At work, go for a walk during your lunch break. You can walk at a relaxed pace.

9.   Use a cordless phone and walk around while talking on the phone.

10.   Move to the sound of the music when a fun song comes on the radio.

11.   Mow the lawn and rake the leaves.

12.   Chop your own firewood.

13.   Park the car a few blocks away and walk the children the rest of the way to
        school.

14.   Shovel the snow by hand at a slow pace.

15.   At the shopping mall, avoid riding the elevators and the escalators.

16.   Wash your car by hand.

17.   At work, deliver your own mail, if possible instead of sending them by
        office mail.

18.   At the office, place supplies in a way in which you need to get up out of your
        chair. If extremely busy, you could always at time place them near you.

19.   When teaching, doing workshops, seminars, in-service training, try moving around.

20.   Walk the dog.

WEIGHT CONTROL AND EXERCISE/PHYSICAL ACTIVITY GO HAND IN HAND: BEFORE YOU START AN EXERCISE PROGRAM, YOU SHOULD FOLLOW CERTAIN RULES:

1.   Consult with your Physician – especially if you were inactive for a long period of time.   He/she will determine whether or not you have any illness, which may restrict you from certain exercise.

2.   Select a suitable exercise program – or sport.

3.   Make your exercise area comfortable.

4.   Proper exercise gear: loose fitting, comfortable clothing, socks, proper sneakers,

5.   Exercise is a building block – start out slow and over a certain period of weeks add more to your program. Goal is to build endurance and stamina. This will strengthen your heart as well as promote good circulation.

6.   Schedule your exercise or sport that you enjoy for the best results. Exercise no less than three times a week. No less than twenty minutes for each workout session.

7.   For the extremely obese – start out with the toning exercise that is provided. You may also walk in place indoors if the weather is bad. As your endurance and stamina increase you may work towards a more strenuous workout.

8.   Stop – If you feel any pain or breathing difficulty it is best to stop the exercise. If you experience pain in either your muscles or joints, you should stop! Usually it

is not necessary to stop if you experience minor soreness. Just monitor your workout; you need to learn your body.

9.   Symptoms – look out for body languages. If you experience pain in the center of your chest, or behind the breastbones, stop. Also, beware of pain that spread to your shoulders, neck, and arms.

Note: If any outbreaks of cold sweat, nausea, shortness of breathe, dizziness and weakness and if any of the symptoms persist, see your physician immediately.

10.   Enjoy – exercise is a vital part of weight reduction and it can be fun. Do not over exert yourself to the point where you are sweating excessively. Do not cause any injury to yourself.

11.   To make exercise fun, you can do the following:

     a.   exercise to music

     b.   exercise while watching television

     c.   exercise with a friend

     d.   jog/walk with a friend

     e.   exercise with a personal trainer

NOTE: REMEMBER TO CONSULT YOUR PHYSICIAN FIRST.

AEROBIC EXERCISE

This form of exercise will enhance cardiovascular fitness and burn fat. It is necessary that the aerobic exercise last at least 20 minutes of continuous exercise.

Dancing can be done by almost everyone. It is a fun way to burn calories and fat. If you are extremely overweight, do not move too much or too fast. You do not want to put too much stress on the joints of the feet, ankles, knees and hips. As you lose more weight, have fun. This is something you can do alone at anytime.

If you are extremely overweight, please note that exercise can help you lose a considerable amount of weight. Check with your physician first.

STEPPING – This exercise can be done when you are unable to go out walking due to bad weather or just do not feel like going outside to exercise. Walking up and down the stairs can be done in your home or any home or at work. Start walking up and down slowly first then, go faster as your weight comes off. This is a good muscle toning exercise. Stair climbing is very strenuous for a very overweight person and should be avoided.

JOGGING and RUNNING – You could eventually jog and run when you become more conditioned. The impact of jogging or running on your lower limbs is about three times your body weight, while the impact of walking is only approximately 1.3 times your body weight. Jogging or running can be dangerous because of the extreme stress on the heart and legs. Check with your physician as always.

- Rope jumping for the very overweight person could cause too much stress on the joints of the feet, ankles, knees and hips. After your weight loss, check your fitness level first.

- Swimming – If you are an average to good swimmer, this is excellent for burning calories and toning every muscle in your body.

OTHER BENEFITS OF PHYSICAL ACTIVITIES ARE:

- Healthier heart, lower risk of heart attack

- Lower blood cholesterol

- More normal blood pressure

- Healthier lungs

- Stronger bones

- More relaxed

- Sleep better

- More energy

DRINKING WATER/EXERCISING:

When you exercise you sweat and lose body fluid. You need to replace the fluids lost. You should drink water before and after you exercise.

Depending on how long you exercise you should also drink water during workouts. If you do workout for a longer period of time, you may want to drink a beverage with carbohydrate.

1. Unsweetened fruit juice (1/2 cup of fruit juice to ½ cup of water).

2. Sport drinks with no more than 10 percent carbohydrate.

Do not drink beverages that are high in sugar when exercising or after workout. You will burn sugar and not fat. With the omission of sugar you will burn fat longer after your workout. **Use this fluid hydration guild during exercise.**

- Drink 2 cups of water two hours before the exercise.

- Drink 2 cups of water about 15 minutes before exercising.

- Drink 1 cup of water every 15 minutes during the workout.

WALK POUNDS AWAY

Walk forward at a leisurely pace. Walk 2 miles in 30 minutes (15 minutes/mile). Walking is an excellent way to lose and maintain weight. It is a type of exercise that is accessible to just about everyone. People that are extremely overweight have extra stress on their joints. Walking is a low-impact activity that goes easy on the joints. Walking is also a good exercise for the beginner. Start out walking at a leisurely pace. Keep it simple. As you lose weight or feel more fit, you may want to advance to brisk walking. People who start out exercising moderately are twice as likely to stick with exercising regimen and increase the intensity in time.

As you advance, there are other exercises or physical activities you can do in place of walking or you may want to still walk plus do other exercises or physical activities on different days.

Example: -running ½ mile in 30 minutes

            -stair walking for 15 minutes

            -bicycling 5 miles in 30 minutes

            -dancing fast for 30 minutes

            -jumping rope for 15 minutes

Always start out with any exercise program moderately and increase the intensity as you become more physically fit. Keeping active is important. A 30-minute brisk walk, four days a week can enable many people to lose a half-pound a week.

Walking can be done by the experienced exerciser or by someone working out for the very first time whether young or older.

Almost everyone can walk even the person that is extremely over weight. It's safe and easy. Just start out slowly until you can walk briskly. If you never build up to brisk walking, slow walking still has many health benefits, but a brisk walk will tone the body more, and walking will increase the blood circulation throughout the body.

BENEFITS OF WALKING

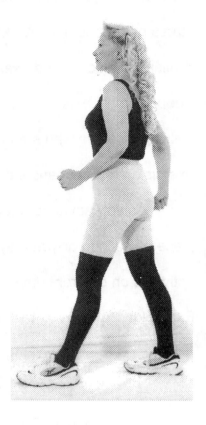

- You will feel better emotionally

- You will have more energy

- Reduce stress

- It will improve your cardiovascular system

- Improved respiratory system

- Improved muscular strength

- Better flexibility

- Best of all promote weight loss and maintenance

WALKING PROGRAM

Walking is said to be the best all around exercise for everyone. The requirement is a good pair of walking shoes.

- Check with your physician first

- Always walk at your own pace

- Time your walks. Start out slowly at first, especially if you are out of shape or extremely overweight

- Start out with short walks and take your time

- As you become more conditioned, you may, if you want, increase your walking to 3 to 4 miles in an hour

- If you do walk briskly, breathe deeply. If you walk briskly for only 20 minutes that is good. You can build up by adding two or more minutes of brisk walking a day until you reach your desired time and past.

- If your heart rate is too fast at first and you get out of breath, stop and check with your doctor. If he or she says everything is good then continue or you may need to slow walk just a little longer before your brisk walk.

- Keep a good full posture throughout your walk

- Look forward, not down at the ground and keep your hips level with your head up.

FLEXIBILITY STRETCHING

Flexibility stretching can be used for warming-up and cooling-down. It is a good working program for the novice and the extremely overweight person. Like walking, it is something that just about anyone can do. It will increase your range of motion as it prepares you in choosing a more advance exercise program as you start to lose weight.

Flexibility stretching is recommended before you do any type of light or heavy strength training. You must start out slowly. The goal of flexibility stretching is for you to start toning the body as you start loosing weight and to assist the beginner or extremely over weight person in improving their daily living through range of motion.

BENEFITS OF FLEXIBILITY STRETCHING

- Start toning the body

- Reduces stress

- Provide you with a sense of well-being

- Improves your ability to function in your life activities

- Improves physical appearance

- Build more self-confidence

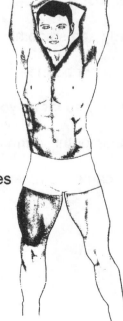

- Relaxes the mind

- Improves circulation

- Improves coordination

- Improves body balance

Once you move to a more advance exercise program, you could still do the strengthening to warm-up before you begin the workout program about 5 minutes and also cool down after you complete your workout.

If you decide not to warm-up, start your exercise program at a slower pace to prevent injury. You should always cool-down by stretching for about 5 minutes.

WHY WARMING-UP / COOLING DOWN?

Warming-up slowly raises the heart rate; helps prevent injuries and warm the muscles.

Cooling-down will do the opposite. Your heart rate will be reduced and your breathing will also slow down.

STRETCHING RULES

1. Go slowly and smoothly, take your time

2. Relax, do not bounce

3. Stretch only as far as you can without pain and hold it for about 5 seconds or so

4. Breathe smoothly during your stretch

Anyone can stretch, large or small, young or old.

BUTTERFLY

Sitting position on the floor, place the bottom of your feet together. Slightly tighten your abdominal muscle as you perform this procedure. Slowly lean forward and touch the floor, pause. Return back to sitting position.

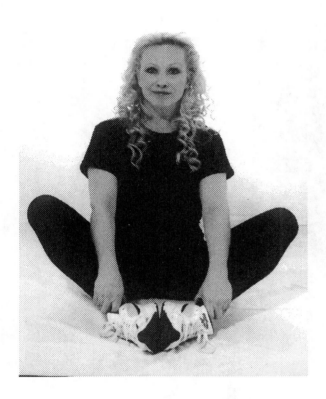

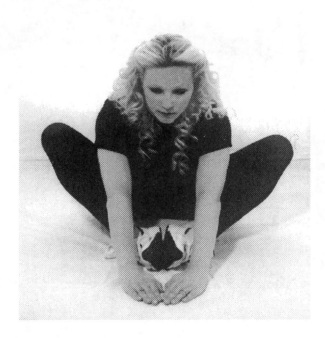

INNER HURDLE STRETCH

Sit with right leg extended and to right diagonal, and left leg bent with left foot touching the right thigh, knee on or near the ground. Slowly reach both hands towards right toe. Hold, and repeat. Reverse position for left leg. Hold. Repeat.

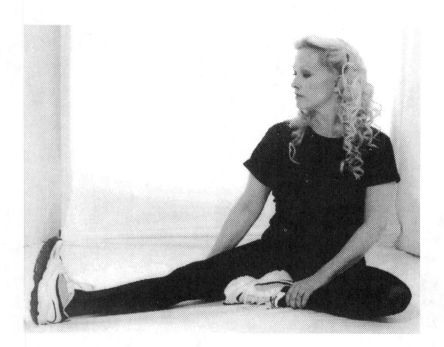

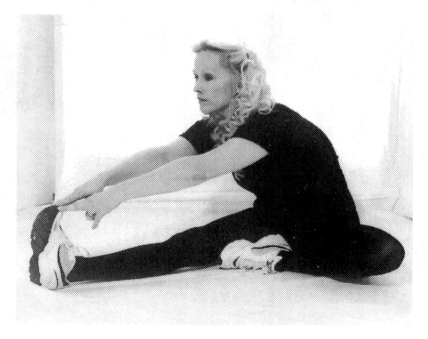

HAMSTRING STRETCH

Start out by laying straight out on the floor on your back. Pull your right knee to your chest and slightly raise your head to your knee, pause. Repeat with your other leg.

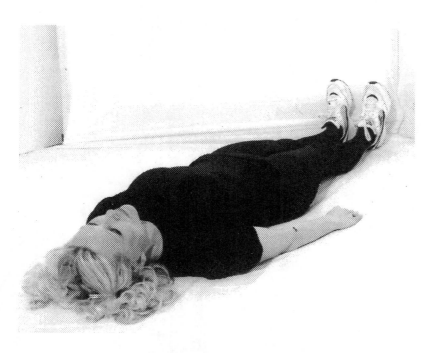

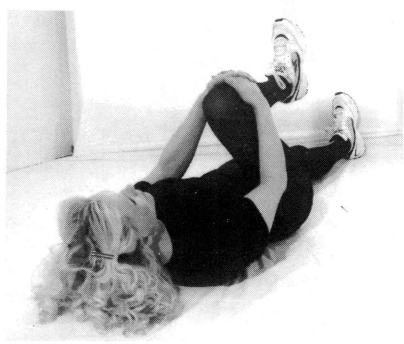

ONE ARM OVER HEAD STRETCH

Place left hand on your hip. Stretch right hand above head, pause. Then change by placing right hand on hip and stretching left hand above your head, pause, and then repeat.

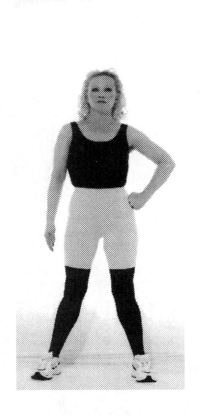
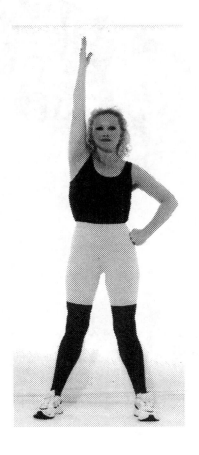

CALF AND SHIN STRETCH

Place right leg forward and left leg out behind in the opposite position. Bend right knee slowly keeping left heel on the floor, pause. Bend left knee while straightening right knee, pause. Repeat it with left leg forward.

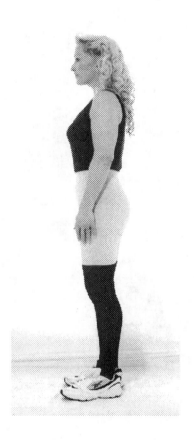

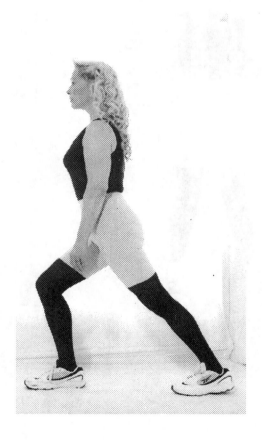

ONE SHOULDER ROLL

Let both arms hang down to your sides. Rotate your right shoulder forward and around.

Then rotate the right shoulder backward and around. Repeat same with the left

shoulder.

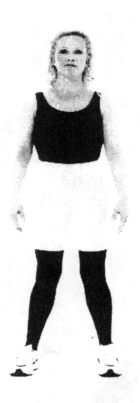

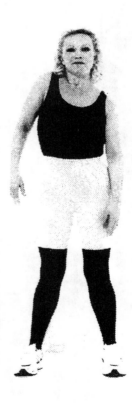

KNEE RAISES

Standing position, raise right knee as high as possible, grasp right knee with both hands. Pull leg up toward your body and keep the back straight, pause. Repeat with left leg.

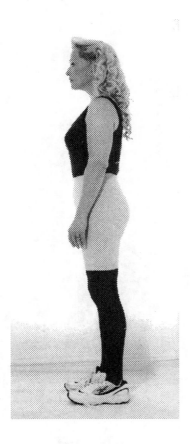
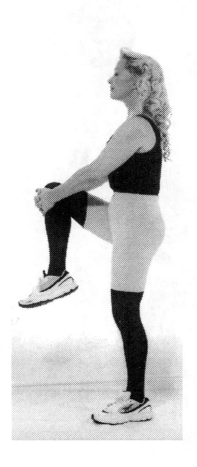

OVERHEAD STRETCH

Extend your arms over your head. Clasp hands together. Bend from waist to the right as your left arm gently stretches to the right side, pause. Return to starting position. Repeat going to the left side.

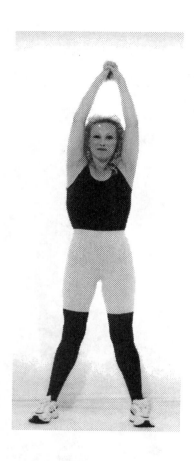

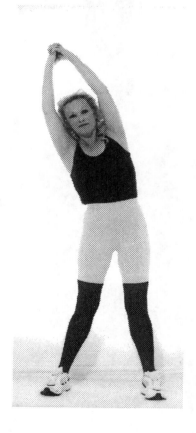

BENDER-OBLIQUES

Standing with the arms bent over your head and with hands on opposite sides, try touching your elbows, bend to the left. Pause, return back to standing position, then bend to the right. Do 10, 15, or 25 reps each side.

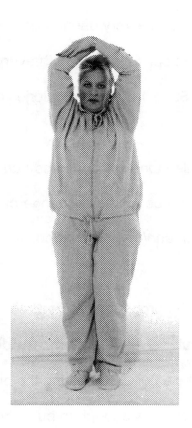

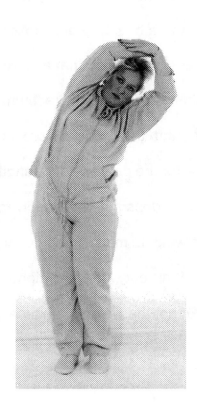

LIGHT STRENGTH TRAINING vs. HEAVY WEIGHT LIFTING FOR WEIGHT LOSS

HEAVY WEIGHT LIFTING:

Heavy weight lifting is not recommended if you want to lose weight. Heavy weight lifting will build muscle (large tissue), which will increase your weight and increase your appetite. This is good for bulking up, increasing body's muscle mass. In the extremely overweight person, heavy weight lifting can be very dangerous. Heavy weight lifting can increase your blood pressure and can cause injury. With every pound of muscle added to your body, you will burn between 50 to 1,000 more calories each day. Muscle also weighs more.

I recommend light strength training. This will also tone the body and burn fat and also help with a healthy weight loss. Heavy weights can be extremely dangerous for the beginner and the people that are extremely overweight and/or out of shape. The use of lightweights or dumbbells is recommended.

Strength training is the process of exercising with progressively heavier resistance for the purpose of strengthening the muscular skeletal system. Building muscle mass does not necessarily mean building muscle bulk. Repeating the process using lightweights many times during an exercise sessions is enough to build firmer muscles. Start out with lightweights and a few repetitions for each exercise. Increase the rep but not the weights. In time you may find it necessary to increase the weights.

BENEFITS OF LIGHT WEIGHT STRENGTH TRAINING

The benefits of strength training like walking are many. You can walk one day and light strength train the next. Light strength training can also be done on days you cannot or do not want to go outdoors to walk for any reason or you can light strength training for your weight loss program only.

BENEFITS OF LIGHT STRENGTH TRAINING

1.   Tones the body

2.   Increase metabolic rate, which will cause you to burn more calories and fats.

3.   Fat stores calories but muscle burns calories. As your body tones the more Calories you will burn automatically throughout the day and night.

4.   Improves your physical appearance.

5.   Improves self-confidence.

6.   Fights osteoporosis.

ONE ARM DUMBBELL ROW

Stand with your right hand on the chair, palm down. Hold dumbbell in the left hand with palm facing in. Let your left hand hang down. Then pull your left arm up until your hand brushes against your waist, pause, then lower the weight slowly back down. If the chair is low, it is okay to slightly bend your knees. You may also tighten your abdominal muscles as you perform this procedure. Do 5, 10, or 15 reps.

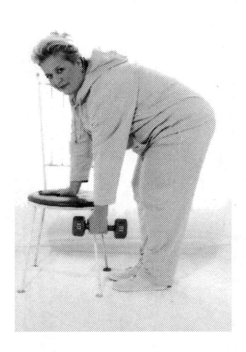

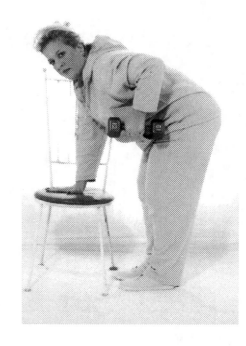

SHOULDER PRESS

Sitting on the chair, with feet on the floor, hold dumbbell in both hands with palms facing toward the front. Bend your elbows; to standing position, upper arms to shoulder height and the dumbbells are at ear level. Tighten your abdominal muscles, and then push the dumbbells up over the head. Then lower the dumbbells back to the ear level. Do 5, 10, or 15 reps.

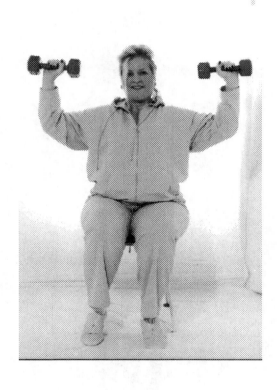

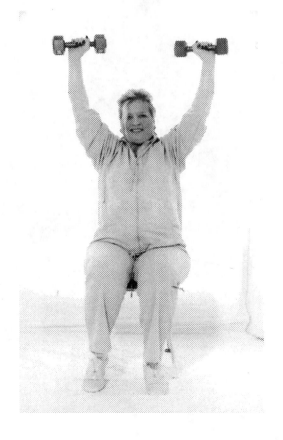

ARM CURL

Sitting position near the edge of the chair. Then, place your feet on the floor a few inches apart. Leaning forward, place your right elbow against the inside of your right thigh. Let the dumbbell hand down toward the floor. Place your left palm on the left thigh. Curl the weight upward to the shoulder and then lower the weight back down. Do 10, 15, or 25 reps.

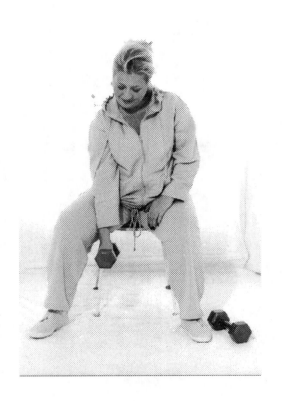

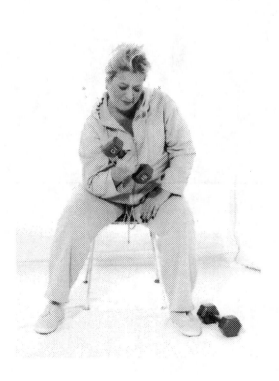

ARM BACK RAISE

Stand with your right hand on the chair, palm down. Hold dumbbell in the left hand with palm facing in. Then bend your left elbow so that your upper arm is parallel to the floor. Hold your elbow close to your waist. Tighten your abdominal muscles. Keep your knees straight or slightly bend your knees. Keep the upper arm still and raise the dumbbell up backward until your arm is parallel to the floor. Slowly bring the arm back parallel to the floor. Do 5 or 10 reps.

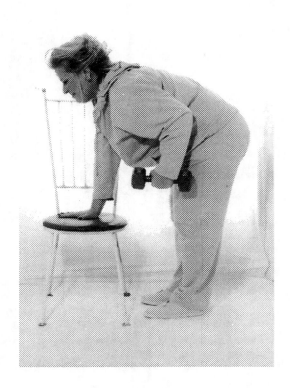

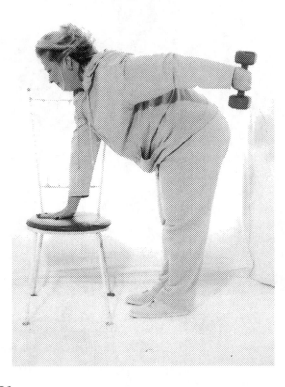

FRONT RAISE

Standing with feet together or slightly apart, grasping weight with both hands, arms straight down, and then raise weight slowly to the chest level. Do not touch the chest; pause, then lower slowly back down. Do 5, 10, or 12 reps.

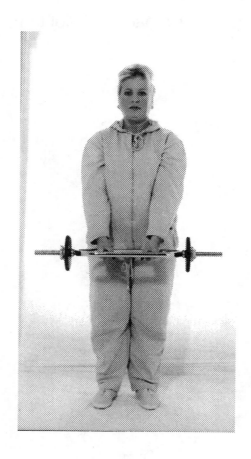

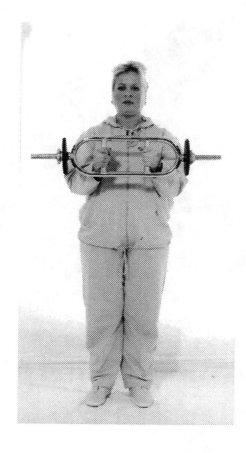

ARM SWINGS

Standing position grasp hold of dumbbell with both hands straight out in front. Then turn and swing to the right pause and then swing your arms to the left. Do 10 to 15 reps.

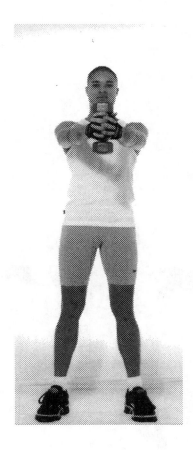

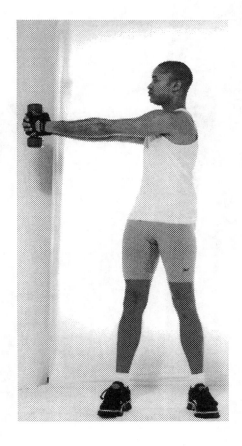

LATERAL ARM RAISE

Hold at your sides a dumbbell in each hand. Keep your arms straight and raise the dumbbells up to your shoulders, then lower dumbbells back to the sides. Repeat 5, 8 or 10 reps.

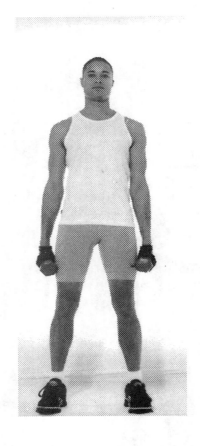

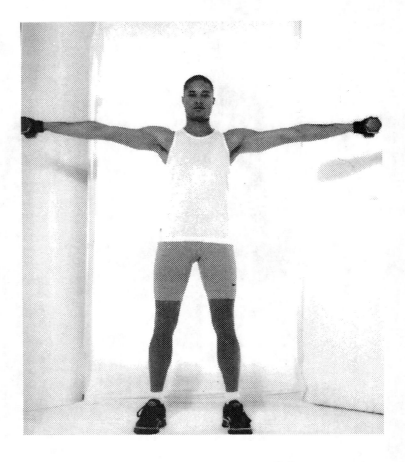

LEG LUNGES

Stand straight up; hold a dumbbell in each hand by your sides. Step out with left leg. Bend knee toward the floor without touching the floor. Push back up with the left foot and return to standing position. Repeat it with right leg and keep alternating to do 10, 15, or 25 reps.

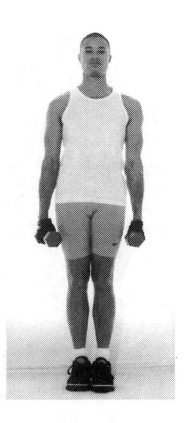

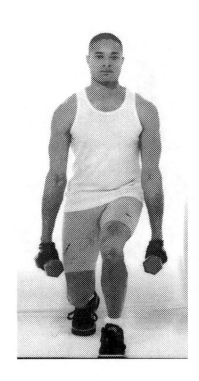

DUMBBELL PRESS

Standing position, grasp and hold dumbbell at neck or head level in each hand. Push the weight upward and then inward over your head. Pause, lower back down slowly and repeat. Do 5, 9, or 12 reps.

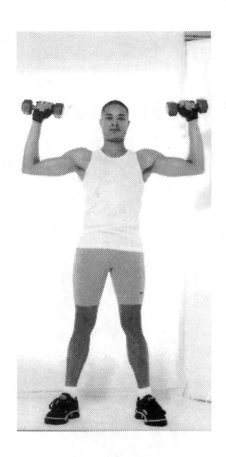

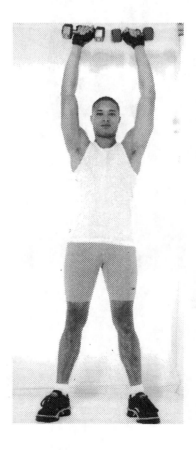

SIDE BEND

Standing position, hold one dumbbell or weight in the right hand, place left hand on hip, or let arm hand straight down, bend down to the left, pause, return back to standing position. Do 5, 10, or 25 reps. Repeat on other side.

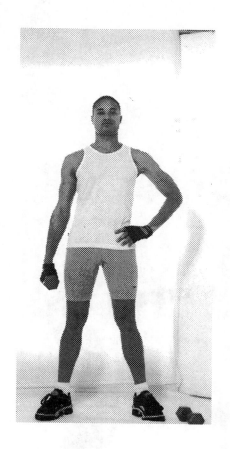

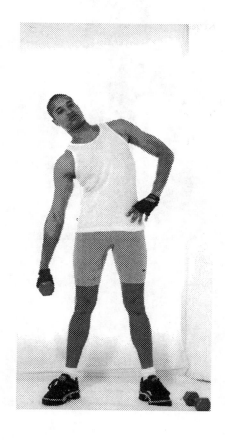

DUMBBELL FRONT RAISE

Standing position, grasp dumbbells in both hands. Hold palms down at your side. Raise your right arm straight out in front to chest level, pause, then lower arm to starting position. Raise left arm. Repeat it for 5, 8, or 12 reps.

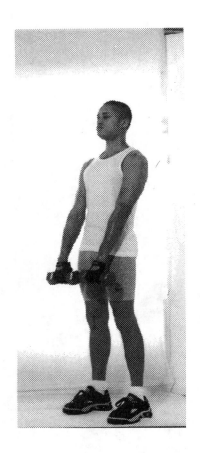

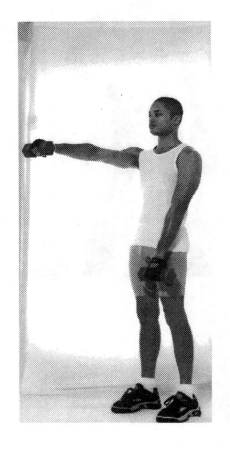

ONE ARM TRICEPS EXTENSIONS

Standing position with one arm at your side, with your other arm hold dumbbell behind the head with arm bent at elbow. Then extend your arm straight overhead. Lower and repeat for 5, 10, or 12 reps. Switch arms.

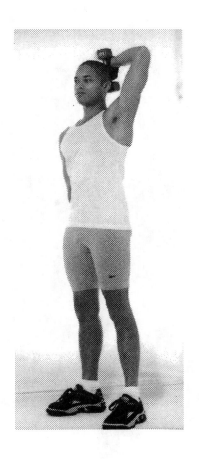

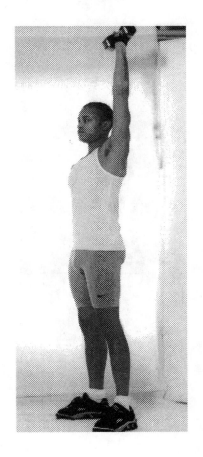

OVERHEAD ARM RAISE

Grasp a dumbbell with both hands, hold behind your neck. Raise overhead and pause. Then, slowly lower the weight back down to starting position. Repeat 5, 8, or 12 reps.

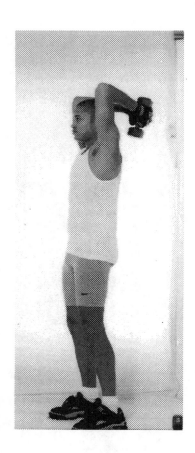

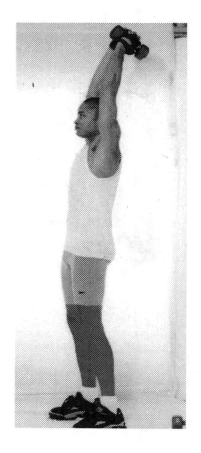

BACK ARM RAISE

Grasp a dumbbell in your left hand, bend forward from your hip so your back is parallel and your knees slightly bent. Hold your left arm up to your waist. Raise the dumbbell out backward, and then bring the weight back to your waist. Do 5, 9, or 12 reps. Repeat with your right hand.

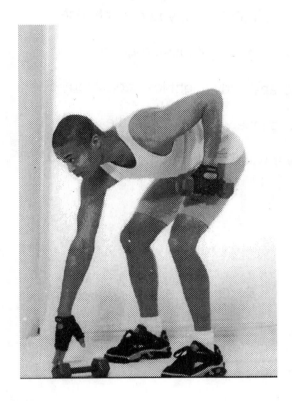

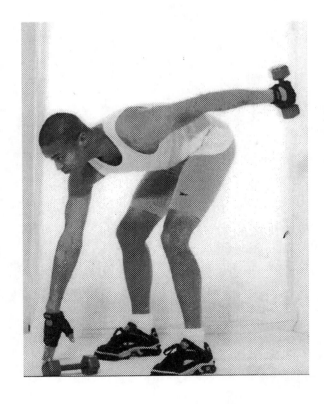

SECTION E – PART II

Everything leading to this section was actually showing you how easy it is to eat healthy and lose weight too. This section will provide you with information that will aid in weight loss and body toning. The information provided can be used as you desire and under your physician's direction. After reviewing Section D Part II, you may choose not to add any of these to your healthy eating/weight loss program. However, I do recommend massage therapy and weight loss coaching. So you see, you do not need will power to lose weight, just a little knowledge will do, okay, a little will power will also help, but it's A, B, C, D, Easy.

Herbal Body Wrap

Herbal Body Wrap is the biggest or greatest missing link in weight loss. No weight loss program should be without it! It's like putting the icing on the cake or having a sandwich without bread or cold cereal without cold milk.

Body Wrap and weight loss will be the marriage of the 21st century. Plastic surgery and drugs have become the weight reduction choice of the 20th century making plastic surgeons and drug companies very rich. There is now for the 21st century a healthy, "all natural" alternative. Herbal Body Wrap and medical nutrition therapy actually removes fat from the body and reduces weight without surgery. You can have a total Body Wrap or you can lose inches on special areas of the body. You can lose inches off the whole body at one time or spot reduction: under arms, legs, abdomen, cheeks, etc.

The Body Wrap was first created to detoxify the body of pollutants, but once the Body Wrap was done, the major discovery was noted that people actually lost inches also. The body became more functional and smooth after each wrap.

Achieving and maintaining a fit, trim body is a continuous process. For this reason you should combine Herbal Body Wrap and nutrition therapy. You will have an even better looking body and you will look and function great! These changes are measured primarily in the area of strength, flexibility and endurance and you will also lose and maintain a healthy body weight.

I like to start my clients off first with medical nutrition therapy by having them start losing weight and after they have lost between 5-15 lbs., then I will start doing Herbal

Body Wrap. You can get rid of fat and inches, between 5-15 inches, from your first Herbal Body Wrap. The fat cells will actually shrink in size.

As I said in the beginning, this is the biggest missing link when it comes to weight lose. I recommend that all my clients be wrapped during the process of their weight loss regimen. Thousands of doctors are using this amazing treatment. I do know that there will be less surgery when it comes to weight loss in the future. Surgery has its place and I am not trying to say that it should not be done, but I do believe that it should be absolutely your last choice.

Human Growth Hormones/Weight Loss - Another missing link to weight loss

As we get older our body cells just get lazy. The cells do not do what they should do. Between the ages of 21 and 61 years old, the body losses up to 80% of this Growth Hormone. These hormones are needed to slow down the aging process, which is also known as anti-aging hormones. There are many good benefits of Human Growth Hormones, but the one that I am mainly concerned with at the present time, is how it relates to weight control and weight loss or to control weight.

Human Growth Hormone stimulates the cells, which causes an increase in metabolism and an increase in the circulation of the liver, which causes the body to automatically lose weight due to the increase in metabolism rate. Researchers are predicting by taking Human Growth Hormones a person may or can live to be up to 130 years of age. Other benefits of Human Growth Hormones are as follows:

1. Weight control (body fat loss)

2. Increase in energy level

3. Feel better

4. Look better (more youthful)

5. Wrinkles are reduced

6. There is an increased muscle tone or strength

7. Improved mood swing

8. Sexual impotency is improved (more frequency)

9. Memory is improved

10. Sleep better at night

11.   Many people report that their gray hair started to turn back to its natural color.

I feel that Growth Hormone is a missing link when it comes to weight loss and maintenance because of the ability of the Growth Hormone to increase the body or cells metabolism which in return burn fat and also increase the body muscle mass percentage to body fat. Human Growth Hormone is not necessary for a healthy weight loss and maintenance. Yes, I do have clients who lose weight without taking Growth Hormones, but it will make so many peoples lives better. Also, just look at the many different added benefits of taking Growth Hormones. You really have nothing to lose but so much to gain to live longer, to look better, to be able to get around at an older age, 100 plus without depending on people to care for you. If we can send a man to the moon, then why can't we do things to improve the quality of health?

Taking Human Growth Hormones along with the other health information provided for a healthy weight loss is so simple. It is probably the simplest regimen that has been provided to you. It is in liquid form. All you need is a few drops under the tongue daily. That's it!

Some Doctors recommend using nature growth hormones cream that can be rubbed directly on the chest. The hormones will absorb through the skin. Avoid taking synthetic growth hormones which can cause problems.

Liquid Vitamins

First is taking vitamins in the form of a pill. Vitamins are needed for the body to function properly. In order for us to get the vitamins that we need, we must eat a variety of foods. Although I do believe that a few people may eat properly in order for them to get the intake that is needed, I also know that there are millions of people who do not. For this reason, I recommend that during weight loss and maintenance that vitamins and mineral supplements are needed. I also recommend that vitamins and minerals should be taken in a liquid form because of the ease of digestion and absorption. Vitamins in the pill form are hard to digest and to absorb because of the high metallic content of the pills, which our bodies were not designed to digest. Many pills are listed as "all natural" but often have added filters and coding that inhibit absorption.

The Physicians Desk Reference show that vitamins and minerals in pill forms are only 10-20% absorbed by the body which means that for every $100 you spend on vitamins, you are basically flushing about 90% of it down the toilet. Liquid vitamins provides about 98% absorption rate because they by-pass the digestive process and go directly into our blood stream and into the cells within a matter of minutes.

All liquid vitamins are not the same. The forms I use and recommend to my clients are from a company who provides a liquid vitamin drink that derives their nutrients from organic sea vegetation. These nutrient-rich vegetables are blended with Aloe Vera and a lot of other tasty, delicious products that provide a nectar flavor. It also contains 120 essential nutrients.

Research has already shown that we cannot eat enough food to get the vitamins and nutrients that we need especially fruits and vegetables. It also shows that the farm soils are depleted of nutrients and the crops are contaminated with pollutants and poisons, which is common knowledge.

Never try to lose weight without the use of some form of vitamins and mineral supplements. For weight maintenance you may need to speak to your healthcare provider. Some forms of vitamins are needed, liquid or pills.

WEIGHT LOSS COACH

A lot of people continue dieting on their own without some form of support. Seek the help of a nutrition counselor or a weight loss coach. Weight loss coaching is new and it is usually done over the phone. The coach and the client would most likely not come face to face. With some of my clients, I meet with them in person, review their needs, and then the follow up is usually done over the phone. At times, I would have clients further away and it is not practical to meet so it is done by phone. After they make their payment by mail, I set a time for the client to call me 4 times a month. If more time is needed, adjust the schedule.

As a weight loss coach, I provide the support needed for eating healthy for life and for weight too.

MASSAGE THERAPY AND WEIGHT CONTROL

Body massage is one of the oldest healing arts, which have been around for centuries and is good for many ailments. Massage not only makes you feel good, but it may help reduce stress, improve blood circulation, lymph circulation, loosen up tight muscles, increase energy, help transport oxygen to tissue and help speed up recovery from injuries. Massage therapy also helps the body eliminate toxins and help save needed energy for other body activities. When energy is saved, more will be used for proper digestion. The energy saved will aide in burning calories. Drink plenty of water after a massage to flush out the toxins from the system. During the massage, lots of fluids and toxins are released and moved throughout the body. If you have chronic illness, or cancer or just had surgery, or if you are taking special medications, check first with your physician before have a body massage. When some extremely obsessed people lose weight too fast, their skin has the tendency to become too flabby. Massage therapy will not only aide with a healthy weight lost, but it will also help keep the body firm.

BATH THERAPY

Twenty minutes in a bath with natural fragrant essential oils will not only soothe and moisturize your skin, it will also help to relax or revitalize your mind. Your mind plays a big part in weight control. Take a relaxing therapy bath to help relax the mind and this may also help control the need to overeat. Essential oils are highly concentrated and are usually diluted in carrier oils for treatment. With the rare exception of lavender and tea tree oil, do not use essential oil full strength. Speak to a professional or an aroma therapist first. They will most likely perform a skin test to check for skin irritation.

HYPNOSIS AND WEIGHT LOSS

There is no magic cure for losing weight. Hypnosis is an alternative treatment that's also been around for centuries and can be helpful for so many conditions. I find that hypnosis works well for people who are under a lot of stress. I am not suggesting that anyone should be hypnotized, but it is a personal choice. If you have any deep emotional problems, consult with your physician first. If you are just generally stressed out about weight loss, it will be worth looking into. What you're looking to do is learn how to relax and hypnosis can often help you prevent continually making unwise food choices and may also prevent repeatedly overeating.

BLUEBERRY LEAF EXTRACT (TEA)

Research has identified two natural compounds that are found in blueberry leaves which are chlorogenic and caffeine acids. The report stated that they may aide in weight loss, The two compounds in blueberry leaves extract may be able to reduce the amount of glucose that is being absorbed, increase the rate in which glucose is metabolized and decreased the amount of glucose that is produced in the liver. This is said to prevent excessive carbohydrates and sugary foods from being converted and stored as body fat. The report also stated that by consuming blueberry leaf tea extract is not a license to overeat carbohydrate rich foods. Remember always to have any nutrient in moderation. You must still follow a healthy meal plan most of the time.

EATING FRESH FRUIT WITH OTHER FOODS

In the first part of the book I recommend that you eat breakfast and the first part of breakfast should consist of fresh fruits. I also stated that it is important to eat fresh fruits also on an empty stomach because fresh fruits require little or no digestion and it is quickly absorbed. The body will immediately receive all the needed vitamins and minerals quickly. I also made a statement throughout the book "never say never" because we can always make exceptions.

You will be given information on why snacking is a necessary part of weight control. I have also provided you with lists of healthy snacking recommendations. I did not want to make my recommendations be in any way considered a fad diet so at times I added fresh fruit combinations with other foods mainly because this is the American way of eating. Example: If you choose to have a few pieces of fresh sliced apples and a few pieces of fresh sliced carrots together, it should not cause a problem because it is only a small portion and you must remember to chew food properly. Just remember, you do not want to eat large portions of fresh fruit with you large regular meal because you do not want the fruit to stay for hours in the stomach digesting because the fruit will spoil.

CALCIUM AND OBESITY

Research showed that increased consumption of dairy products high in calcium can cause weight reduction and total body fat in adults and children. A healthier meal plan higher in calcium and lower-fat dairy products may help increase the amount of dietary fat being burned. The study reported the following:

1. Children – For every 300 mg of increased calcium consumed there was approximately 2 pounds decreased in body fat.

2. Adults – For every 300 mg of increased dietary calcium, there was approximately 5.5 to 6.6 decreased in total body weight.

MEAT PROTEIN AND WEIGHT CONTROL

A protein-based meal will allow you to burn more calories. You will burn more calories because digestion of protein requires more energy than carbohydrate or fats. When you consume a meal that contains protein (meat), you will burn about 600 more calories. Although eating protein will boost the metabolism and help control your weight, only a small amount is needed to do the job. Rule of thumb, you do not need any more than 6 oz. of flesh protein for the day. Avoid overloading on protein the same as overloading on carbs. Review page 102 for other sources of proteins, other than meat protein.

CARBOHYDRATE LOVERS AND WEIGHT CONTROL

For people who crave carbohydrates, it is not necessary to avoid pasta, rice, potatoes, etc. The key is to eat carbohydrates with a protein or grain. Protein and grain foods are higher in fiber and is a natural appetite suppressive. A combination of protein and grain will fill you up and help prevent the early onset of hunger. Eating carbohydrate foods, like any other nutrients, does not cause obesity. Overloading on any food group must be avoided. So, enjoy your pasta etc. in moderation, but try to eat more carbs that are higher in fiber along with lower-fat flesh protein foods. Higher fiber foods will also prevent the early on-set of hunger which will help prevent overeating, and as said before, the protein combination meal will also speed up the metabolism which will cause more calories to be burned.

CHEWING GUM FOR WEIGH LOSS

A person can burn extra calories just by chewing gum. Chewing gum is said to burn an additional 11 calories per hour. If you do not make any changes in your daily activities or perform any other exercises but walking and chewing gum at the same time for about one hour, you can lose about 10 pounds of body fat in a year.

FIDGETING

I have written something about keeping active and constantly be on the move as much as possible. It is already proven that most people with sedentary lifestyles and the so-called "couch potato" are usually heavier than the more active person.

Researchers used the term fidgety for those people who are always or are constantly moving and they are usually thinner. Report states try to keep moving at all times to help keep the metabolism raised. This will help burn more body fats and total calories. The research is actually saying what I have been telling for years.

Example: If your office or at home when working, make sure you set the flow in a way that you will be constantly moving to get the items you need to do your work.

Researchers also stated that while sitting down at your desk, talking on the phone, etc., tap your feet, tap your fingers, move around and just keep on moving; you will be surprised how much weight you've lost at the end of the year.

TAI CHI EXERCISE

Exercise can be fun. Tai chi type of exercise has been done by Asians for centuries. It can help streamline the body over time and provide the body with a feeling of balance, and it can also help control overeating. This type of exercise can be done by the obese individual because it is slow moving and during weight loss, it can also help tone the body. This type of exercise will also help to burn additional calories and increase the metabolism and help burn extra body fat. Always consult your physician first.

SURGERY

I do not recommend surgery for weight loss if possible. Like anything else, surgery has it's place for treating many conditions as well as weight loss. But, surgery should be the absolutely last resort. In order for you to have surgery for weight loss, doctors will require you to meet certain criteria. For instance, morbid obesity, life and death situation, or 100 lbs. over your ideal body weight. Sometimes after you lose the weight even with exercising, your body may be extremely flabby and have excess fat deposits in certain areas. This condition may need to be corrected with surgery. This decision should be made by you and your physician.

FENNEL TEA

It has been reported that a female weighing about 210 lbs. lost 70 lbs. from drinking fennel tea. Try it, you will never know, it may work for you. Follow a healthy meal plan and drink four cups of fennel tea daily. The recommendation was to drink one cup before breakfast, one cup for morning break or snack, one cup before dinner and one cup just before bed. You can also try taking powdered fennel seed capsules instead.

APPLE CIDER VINEGAR

Apple cider vinegar is said to contain powerful enzymes that can actually dissolve solid fat in the body and wash it right out of the system. It was said to be so powerful that even a small amount of apple cider vinegar will break up the built up fat in the cell tissues shortly after consumed. It has been suggested to add two tablespoons of apple cider vinegar to a glass of vegetable or fruit juice. I recommend that you may want to try making your own fresh vegetable or fruit juice. Use a juicer to make fresh carrot, celery, tomato or a blend of vegetable or fruit juice. Mix in two tablespoons of apple cider vinegar per glass just before serving.

*Note: for any program or meal plan to work, you need to give it time.

INDEX

A

Acid balance – 31
Activities (in place of eating) - 84, 90
Activity, lack of – 88
Advanced workout – 197
Aerobic exercise – 200
Alkaline balance – 31
Alpha linolenic – 95
Alpha linolenic acid – 95
Alpha/Omega – 3 (fatty acid) – 95
Apple cider vinegar – 246
Arroz con pollo – 182
Arthritis – 6
Asparagus soup – 183
Avocado dip – 177

B

Bacon dip – 180
Bag breakfast – 59
Baking with oil – 166
Barbecuing – 157, 172
Bath therapy – 239
Bean salad – 137
Beef seasoning – 169
Beef with eggplant – 184
Behavior modification – 82, 90
Behavior modification techniques - 82, 86
Benefits of physical activities - 201
Benefits of stretching – 205
Binge eating – 13, 14
Blueberry leaf extract (tea) – 241
Body fat – 9
Brain – 6
Breaded vegetable (main dish) 154
Breakfast – 25, 27, 36
Broiling – 156
Burn fat and calories – 86

C

Calcium and obesity – 242
Carbohydrate – 2
Carbohydrate, complex – 106, 107, 150
Carbohydrate lovers and weight control – 243
Carbohydrate source – 105
Cardia – 38
Carrot salad – 138
Chewing gum for weight loss - 244
Chicken seasoning – 170
Chicken with rice – 182
Chili con carne – 184
Chitterlings, saturated – 99

Cholesterol – 97, 104, 105
Chopped chicken liver – 178
Circulatory system – 5
Clam dip – 176
Coconut, saturated – 99
Cole slaw – 137
Colon – 6
Combination foods – 159
Consomme with oxtails – 182
Control total calories – 166
Cooking healthy – 154, 155
Cooking low fat – 143
Cooking methods – 158
Cooking tips – 144
Corn dip – 175
Cream cheese topping, strawberry – 178

D

Defatting ground beef – 157
Defatting recipes – 166
Dessert – 42, 117
Diabetes – 5
Diet – 11, 15, 23
Dietary fat – 2
Dietitian – 17
Dinner – 47, 86
Dipper – fruit – 140
　　　　healthy – 172
　　　　starch – 140
　　　　vegetables – 139
Dips, reduced fat – 172

E

Eat to lose weight – 23
Eating – 52, 61
Eating for the wrong reason – 89
Eating healthy – 20, 51
Eating low fat – 143
EFA – 95
Eggs, seasoning – 170
Emotional problems – 16
Exercise – 194, 196, 197, 200, 207
Exercise rules – 199
Exercising/water – 202

F

Fat – 91, 94, 100
Fat burning foods – 107
Fat craving – 22
Fat free foods – 129, 130
Fat source – 93
Fatty acids – 96

Female obesity – 7
Fennel tea – 246
Fiber – 67, 77
Fidgeting – 244
Fish – 99
Food – 53
Food group – 119
    Bread – 123
    Fruit – 126, 127
    Meat – 119 - 122
    Milk - 122
    Vegetables – 125
Food labels – 113
Food list, allowed, to avoid - 53 – 58
Food prep - 160
Frozen dinner replacement – 60
Fruit – 25, 28
Fruit and weight control – 31
Fruit dip – 175
Fruit salad – 138-139

G
Gallbladder – 6
Glandular – 88
Gout – 6
Gravy, low fat – 179
Grilling – 156
Guacamole dip – 177

H
Ham & pea soup – 185
Healthy eating – 61, 91
Healthy cooking – 154
Heart – 5
Herbal body wrap – 233
High fat food – 100
Human growth hormones – 235
Hunger – 2, 52
Hydrate – 32
Hydrogenated fat - 97
Hypnosis – 240

I
Italian herbs seasoning – 170
Italian style yogurt dip – 173

J
Jogging – 201

K
Kidneys – 5

L
LA – 95
Lamb seasoning – 169
Lean meat – 144

Lean meat cooking – 144–146
Lean muscle tissue – 23
Lean pork – 147-148
Light strength training – 216
Light weight exercises – 218, 231
Light weight training – 217
Linolenic acid – 95
Liquid vitamins – 237
LNA – 95
Low calorie – 23, 62
Low fat cooking – 143-149
Low fat eating – 143
Low fat frying – 143
Lunch – 44
Lungs – 6

M
Macaroni salad – 138
Maintenance – 111
Male obesity – 7
Marinade sauce – 172
Massage therapy – 139
Meal schedule – 35
Measurement and weight – 16
Meat protein and weight control – 243
Meat seasoning – 171
Metabolic rate – 4
Microwave, low fat cooking – 158
Monounsaturated – 95
Muscle tissue lean – 23

N
No fat salad dressing – 174
Nutrients – 90, 91, 101, 104
Nutrition counselor – 17
Nutritionist – 17
Nuts – 129

O
Obesity - 7, 8
Obesity cause – 87, 88
Obesity/death – 8
Obesity/hazards – 5
Oil – 96, 129
Oil conversion chart – 166
Omega 3 fatty acids – 99, 100
Onion dip – 179
Oriental sauce – 172
Osteoporosis – 95
Overeating – 40, 85, 88

P
Pancreas – 6
Paprika blend - 171
Pasta salad – 138, 152
Pesto dip – 180

Physical activities – 194, 196, 198, 201
Physician – 16
Poaching – 156
Polyunsaturated fat – 95
Pork – 170
Portion size – 66
Potato baked – 151
Potato mashed - 150
Potato salad - 138
Potato tomato soup – 183
Power of fruit – 28
Pre-boiled - 158
Pre-meal – 25, 42, 59, 187
Pregnancy – 7
Protein – 101
Protein source – 102
Psychiatrist – 16
Psychologist – 16

Q
Quick fix – 81

R
Raise metabolism – 61
Recipe makeover – 180
Recipe, changing – 150, 163, 164, 165
Recipes – 160, 161, 162, 164, 166, 168
Regaining weigh – 89
Running - 201

S
Salads – 136
Saturated fats – 99
Sauce – 153
Sauce, keeping it healthy – 153
Sausage, macaroni dinner – 181
Sauteing – 156
Seasoning – 49, 131, 169, 170
Seasoning salt – 171
Set point – 4, 195
Shopping – 111, 115, 140
Shopping advanced – 119, 140
Shopping bigger – 115, 118
Shrimp dip – 179
Sickness and exercise – 20
Simmering – 156-157
Skipping breakfast – 27
Smaller meals – 61
Smart balance – 49
Snacking – 42, 61, 62, 187
Snacking and sleeping – 66
Sour cream dip – 175, 176
Sour cream homemade – 174
Spicy seasoning – 171
Spinach dip – 175
Spraying pan – 156

Spraying pan non-stick cooking – 156
Splenda – 49
Steam basket – 158
Stepping exercises – 201
Stomach – 6
Stretching – 205, 206
Stretching exercises – 207-215
Sugar – 77 – 79
Surgery – 6, 245

T
Tai-Chi exercise – 245
Teenagers – 15
Toppings, healthy – 133-135
Toppings, homemade – 187
Trans-fatty acids – 98
Trim the fat – 145
Turkey – 148

U
Unsaturated fat – 95

V
Veal, seasoning – 169
Vegetable seasoning – 171
Vegetable omelet – 186
Vegetable oil for cooking an seasoning – 165
Vegetable dippers – 139
Vegetable oils – 96, 129
Vegetable, frozen – 136
Vinaigrette dressing – 187, 193

W
Walking – 202-204
Walking program – 204
Warm up – 206
Water – 2, 25, 32, 33, 34, 202
Weight – 28, 31, 32, 34
Weight control – 97, 160
Weight control and exercise – 199
Weight gain – 8, 13
Weight lifting for weight loss – 216
Weight loss – 13, 16, 19, 32, 33, 61, 67, 77, 91, 111
Weight loss coach – 238
Weight maintenance – 77, 111
Weight (regaining) - 89
Weighing yourself – 15
Will power – 2

X

Y
Yogurt dip – 173, 176
Z

Nutritionist – John Mayes, RD CDN LNHA

One of my goals was to write a book dealing with weight loss. Years ago I had started writing a book and almost completed it several times, got frustrated and set it aside, put away never to be completed.

As a nutritionist, my main goal was to show people how to lose weight and keep it off. If you notice, most of the books written about weight loss and maintenance are not written by graduate nutritionists from a qualified institution. So who's better to write a book on weight loss but an expert in the field of nutrition. My frustration is due to the fact that every time I believe that I could solve the weight loss problem, something new would come up and there I go, back to the drawing board. For years, I have been telling my colleagues and patients that dieting just does not work and there is no quick fix to this very day.

I decided to approach weight loss and maintenance in a different perspective. Everyone is spending so much time on losing weight and the one that's successful on weight loss, an extremely high percentage of them regain the weight back in a relatively short period of time. This book is all about eating healthy for life most of the time, and if you follow what I mapped out, you will be eating healthier for total health and the side effect will be permanent weight loss and maintenance. Some willpower may be required, but a little knowledge is the key.

JOHN MAYES, RD CDN LNHA

Member:

* The American Dietetic Association – Registration

* The University of the State of New York – Certified Dietitian – Nutritionist

* State of New York Department of Health – License Nursing Home Administrator